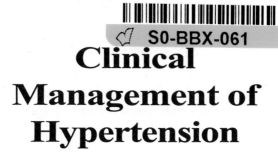

S0-BBX-061

Clinical Management of Hypertension

Second Edition

Marvin Moser, MD, FACP

Clinical Professor of Medicine,
Yale University School of Medicine;
Senior Medical Consultant,
National High Blood Pressure Education Program,
National Heart, Lung and Blood Institute;
Emeritus Chief of Cardiology,
White Plains Hospital Medical Center,
White Plains, New York

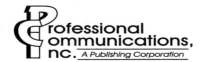

Professional Communications, Inc. *A Publishing Corporation*

DEDICATION

To the many hundreds of researchers and clinicians whose efforts have improved the management of hypertension and have helped to reduce morbidity and mortality from cardiovascular disease.

To the thousands of individuals involved in the National High Blood Pressure Education Program who have charted the course for better care of hypertensive vascular disease.

And to the memory of Herbert Langford, Walter Kirkendall and Irvine Page, three colleagues and friends who helped define and clarify the hypertension "mosaic."

ACKNOWLEDGMENT

I am indebted to Phyllis Freeny for her help in putting this manuscript into its final form;

To Adrienne Cramer, my research associate, for her help in all of our endeavors over the past 20 plus years; and

Finally, to the Westchester Hypertension Foundation for research support.

TABLE OF CONTENTS

TABLES

FIGURES

About the Author

Dr. Moser has been the senior medical consultant to the National High Blood Pressure Education Program of the National Heart, Lung and Blood Institute since 1974. He was chairman of the first Joint National Committee on the Detection, Evaluation and Treatment of High Blood Pressure (JNC) in 1977, Vice-Chairman of the committee in 1980 and has been a member of each of the other four JNCs. He is the author of more than 350 scientific papers and nine books, the latest being *Myths, Misconceptions and Heroics, the Story of the Treatment of Hypertension* from the 1930s, published in 1997.

Preface to 2nd Edition

Since publication of the first edition of *Clinical Management of Hypertension* approximately 1 year ago, several important studies relating to the treatment of this disease have been concluded. In addition, data on some of the newer antihypertensive drugs, including combination therapies, have been expanded.

Importantly, the report of the Sixth Joint National Committee (JNC-VI) on the Detection, Evaluation and Treatment of Hypertension has been published. This second edition of *Clinical Management of Hypertension* incorporates data from this report as well as other studies dealing with the management of hypertension.

1 Introduction

The management of hypertension has undergone a profound change since the 1940s and 1950s when many physicians were still not convinced that an elevated blood pressure greatly increased the risk of cardiovascular disease. Treatment of hypertension was primitive and consisted of a rigid low-sodium diet that few people could follow, mutilative surgeries (such as sympathectomy or bilateral adrenalectomy), and a few medications whose toxic effects were deterrents to their widespread use. Studies in the late 1940s had established that if blood pressure could be lowered in severe or malignant hypertension and sustained at lower levels, many strokes and cases of heart failure could be prevented and survival increased. Physicians began to treat patients with less severe hypertension in the 1960s to 1980s as data from several large clinical trials confirmed that even slight elevations of pressure above an arbitrary limit of 140/90 mm Hg increased cardiovascular risk, and that lowering pressures from these levels would decrease complications.

This handbook is not intended as a complete textbook on hypertension; for that, the reader is referred to standard textbooks. It will, however, highlight some of the recent advances in treatment and discuss a program that includes not only lifestyle interventions, but also the use of available medications.

The program outlined represents our present approach to management, an approach that we have found to be practical and successful as it has evolved over the past 40 years. Not all medications within each class of drugs are discussed; choice of therapy is obviously an individual one, but we have made specific suggestions as to when and how we believe certain therapies should be used. Much of the data in the Fifth and Sixth Joint National Committee Reports on Detection, Evaluation and Treatment of High Blood Pressure, which were published in the *Archives of Internal Medicine* in 1993 and 1997, will be reviewed and critiqued. Specific details for the treatment of malignant or accelerated hypertension, hypertension in pregnancy, etc. can be found in these reports.

We hope that this brief review of hypertension management will be of value to the primary-care physician and internist in the treatment of hypertensive patients.

2 Diagnosis

As late as the 1950s and 1960s, some physicians believed that an elevated blood pressure was necessary to provide an adequate blood supply to vital organs as people aged. Following the landmark Framingham Study and other epidemiologic studies (ie, Tecumseh, LA County), it became obvious, however, that as blood pressure increases even from levels of 110-115/75-80 mm Hg, the risk for cardiovascular events increases. Risk increases more dramatically when pressures rise above 140/90 mm Hg. Therefore, an arbitrary number was assigned as a definition of hypertension: 140/90 mm Hg or above. Later, it became apparent that lowering pressure from these levels decreases the incidence of cardiovascular events.

Classification of Hypertension

For many years, it was also believed that diastolic blood pressure was more important than systolic in defining future cardiovascular risk. More recent data however, have established that elevated systolic pressure may increase risk more than comparatively elevated diastolic pressure. For example, in the Multiple Risk Factor Intervention Trial (MRFIT), where more than 300,000 men were tracked, systolic blood pressure levels of 150 to 159 mm Hg conferred a greater relative risk for coronary heart disease events than diastolic levels of 95 to 100 mm Hg (Figure 2.1).

In addition, it has been clearly established that isolated systolic hypertension, defined in some countries as 160 mm Hg systolic with 90 mm Hg or below diastolic, also increases risk not only for stroke and

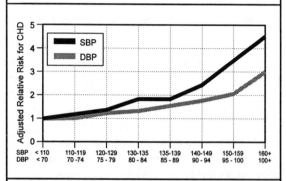
congestive heart failure, but for coronary heart disease events as well. Of importance is the fact that lowering blood pressures from these levels decreases morbidity and mortality. Recent data have also established that isolated *borderline* systolic hypertension (ie, blood pressures of 140 to 159 mm Hg systolic with a diastolic below 90 mm Hg) also significantly increases risk for cardiovascular events and for the future development of more severe hypertension. Patients with these levels of pressures should be treated with lifestyle modifications. If systolic blood pressure remains above 145 to 150 mm Hg, medication may be tried. There is no proof as yet that morbidity or mortality is reduced in these patients by specific treatment, but if blood pressure can be lowered with a simple

regimen without side effects, it is probably worthwhile.

The Fifth Joint National Committee (JNC-V) redefined hypertension to conform to newer data defining risk. The designations of mild, moderate and severe hypertension were changed to the following:

- Stage I: 140-159/90-99 mm Hg
- Stage II: 160-179/100-109 mm Hg
- Stage III: 180-209/110-119 mm Hg
- Stage IV: ≥ 210 mm Hg/≥ 120 mm Hg

A category of high-normal was defined, with diastolic pressures of 80 to 89 mm Hg, and systolic pressures of 130 to 139 mm Hg. This designation did not suggest that patients who have these pressures should be vigorously treated; rather, they should be followed because they are at greater risk for cardiovascular disease than patients with lower pressures, especially if they have other risk factors for heart disease, ie, diabetes, hyperlipidemia, history of smoking, etc.

The Sixth Joint National Committee again changed levels of blood pressures considered optimal, normal or high normal and eliminated the Stage IV classification. Severe hypertension is relatively rare and the approach to therapy is similar at blood pressures of 180-190/100 mm Hg or 210/120 mm Hg except for patients with acute symptoms, ie, hypertensive urgencies or emergencies. The new classification reflects additional data (Table 2.1)

The diagnosis of hypertension should not be made on one visit, unless pressures are above 160-170/105-110 mm Hg; treatment is clearly indicated in these instances. Pressures at levels lower than these should be checked several times over a 3- to 6-month period as lifestyle modifications are made (see Section 3, *Lifestyle Modifications*). In our experience, pressures return toward normal levels in approximately 20% to 25% of subjects with Stage I hypertension.

TABLE 2.1 — JNC-VI CLASSIFICATION OF BLOOD PRESSURE FOR ADULTS AGE 18 YEARS AND OLDER			
Category	Systolic (mm Hg)		Diastolic (mm Hg)
Optimal	< 120	and	< 80
Normal	< 130	and	< 85
High-normal	130-139	or	85-89
Hypertension			
Stage I*	140-159	or	90-99
Stage II*	160-179	or	100-109
Stage III*	≥ 180	or	≥ 110

* Based on the average of two or more readings taken at each of two or more visits after an initial screening.

In addition to classifying stages of hypertension on the basis of average blood pressure levels, clinicians should specify presence or absence of target organ disease and additional risk factors. This specificity is important for risk classification and treatment.

JNC-VI. *Arch Intern Med*. In press.

"White-Coat" Hypertension

There are approximately 20% of people whose pressures are higher in a doctor's office than at home. These patients should not be ignored. They may already have physiologic changes when compared to people whose pressures are normal at home *and* in a doctor's office:

- Vascular resistance tends to be increased.
- There may be evidence of left ventricular diastolic dysfunction.

- Chemically, they resemble patients with early hypertension, ie, there is evidence of increased insulin resistance, and lipid levels tend to be higher.
- More patients with "white coat" hypertension are obese and have diabetes than normotensive (in office and at home) individuals. **2**

The question arises, should patients with "white-coat" or "office" hypertension undergo ambulatory blood pressure monitoring or should decisions be made on the basis of office readings or, in some cases, home blood pressure recordings?

Based on available data and our own experience, we believe that office blood pressures are reliable indicators of outcome. If these pressures are not reduced to normal levels (< 140/90 mm Hg) during the 3- to 6-month period of observation, the patient should be treated with medication, regardless of the level of home or worksite pressures.

Ambulatory Blood Pressure Monitoring

It should be pointed out that all of the data upon which we base our estimates of risk were accumulated from casual blood pressure readings taken in an office or clinic. The higher the "casual pressure," the greater the risk of a cardiovascular event. It should also be remembered that the data upon which we estimate benefit of treatment are also based on casual pressures. In clinical trials such as the Systolic Hypertension in the Elderly Program (SHEP) and the Hypertension Detection and Follow-up Program (HDFP), pressures were taken in an office or clinic every 3 to 4 months; patients with the lowest pressures had the best outcome.

Ambulatory blood pressure monitoring has contributed information on the circadian rhythm of blood pressure, establishing that blood pressure decreases during sleeping hours and increases within an hour or two of arousal in the morning. It has also helped to define a certain subset of patients whose pressures do not decrease from 2 AM to 6 AM. These so-called "non-dippers" are more likely to have left ventricular hypertrophy. This phenomenon is more common in the Black population.

Although ambulatory monitoring has proved to be an interesting research tool and is also useful in establishing the duration of action of new drugs, it was not recommended by the JNC-V or JNC-VI as a routine procedure in the initial evaluation of the hypertensive patient. We agree with this recommendation and do not believe that the expense of this procedure is justified at this time. Nor do we believe that the data provided influence therapeutic decisions in the vast majority of patients.

Some patients want to know their blood pressure. In these cases, or in situations where symptoms are confusing (eg, dizziness—is this the result of pressures that are too high or too low?), pressures can be taken at home with an inexpensive sphygmomanometer. A series of readings over time may actually provide more information than one 24-hour recording.

Diagnostic Evaluation

The JNC-V and JNC-VI have suggested a relatively inexpensive and simple diagnostic evaluation. This includes a careful history and physical examination and blood chemistries that help to rule out not only renal failure but also a possible secondary cause of hypertension (eg, primary aldosteronism), by checking serum potassium levels. A lipid profile is also suggested (Table 2.2). These recommendations have not changed significantly since the first JNC report in 1977.

TABLE 2.2 — SUGGESTED INITIAL EVALUATION FOR THE PATIENT WITH HYPERTENSION

- History and physical examination
- Urinalysis
- Chemical profile, including lipids
- Electrocardiogram
- Renin, catecholamines and aldosterone levels are NOT recommended in the initial evaluation unless there are specific clinical clues to indicate them

Data from: JNC-V. *Arch Intern Med.* 1993;153:154-183 and JNC-VI. *Arch Intern Med.* In press.

An Echocardiogram — Should It Be Done as a Routine Procedure?

An electrocardiogram was suggested by the JNC-V and JNC-VI to detect arrhythmias and evidence of ischemic heart disease. An echocardiogram was not recommended as a routine procedure for the following reasons: It was recognized that an echocardiogram is a more sensitive indicator of left ventricular hypertrophy than an electrocardiogram. However, patients whose blood pressures remain above 140/90 mm Hg after several recordings and several months of lifestyle intervention should have their pressure lowered with medication, whether or not left ventricular hypertrophy is present. In addition, although some investigators believed for many years that the presence or absence of left ventricular hypertrophy could be used as a guide for initial therapy, it has now been demonstrated in several recent studies that all of the drugs suggested as possible first-step therapy, ie, the β-blockers, calcium channel blockers, ACE inhibitors, and diuretics will reverse left ventricular hypertrophy if blood pressure is lowered. It is, therefore, unnecessary to order an echocardiogram in the initial evaluation of the hypertensive patient unless there is another specific indication for this procedure.

Additional studies over and above those recommended in Table 2.1 may be necessary in:

- Patients with hypertension who are below the age of 15
- Elderly patients (> 65 years of age) with recent onset of moderately severe or severe hypertension
- Individuals with persistent elevations of blood pressure after triple-drug therapy
- People with hypertension and symptoms of headache, unusual patterns of sweating and palpitations.

In these instances, procedures to rule out renovascular disease, primary aldosteronism or pheochromocytoma should be undertaken. Details of these procedures can be found in any standard textbook on hypertension.

Summary

Hypertensive patients should be approached with a confident attitude that the complications that used to occur in many patients can be prevented. The diagnostic evaluation is relatively simple in the majority of cases. If lifestyle modifications are unsuccessful in lowering blood pressure, appropriate pharmacologic therapy will reduce blood pressure in more than 75% to 80% of patients, and will reduce morbidity and mortality.

3

Lifestyle Modifications

If blood pressures are higher than 140/90 mm Hg during an initial examination, a diagnosis of hypertension is not justified, but some form of intervention is probably indicated. These interventions should be carried out and another visit scheduled for a blood pressure check and confirmation of the diagnosis. If blood pressure is higher than 160-170/100-105 mm Hg, specific therapy is probably indicated.

There are numerous lifestyle modifications advocated for lowering blood pressure. Many of them, however, may not be effective. Although everyone would like to be in charge of their own destiny and manage a disease process without the use of medication or other treatments, this is often not possible in the management of hypertension. A list of possible lifestyle changes is shown in Table 3.1.

Weight Loss

A high percentage of people with elevated blood pressure are obese. It is well known that obesity predisposes people to hypertension and diabetes. Upper body or abdominal obesity (more common in men), so-called android or apple-shaped obesity, is more frequently associated with dyslipidemia, diabetes and elevated blood pressure than obesity involving the buttocks or thighs. The latter is more common in women, and is called gynecoid or pear-shaped obesity. The most effective method to possibly *prevent* the development of hypertension in normotensive individuals or to lower blood pressure in hypertensive individuals is to maintain normal weight or, if obese, to lose weight. Many patients do not know what their ideal weight should be. Table 3.2 describes how to estimate ideal weight.

TABLE 3.1 — LIFESTYLE MODIFICATIONS FOR CONTROL OF HYPERTENSION AND/OR OVERALL CARDIOVASCULAR RISK

- Weight loss, if overweight*
- Reduction of sodium intake to less than 100 mmol/day (2.4 g of sodium or approximately 6 g of sodium chloride)*
- Limiting alcohol intake to < 1 oz/day of ethanol (24 oz of beer, or 10 oz of wine, or 2 oz of 100 proof whiskey); approximately one half of these amounts for women and thin people
- Cessation of smoking and reduction of dietary saturated fat and cholesterol for overall cardiovascular health; reduced fat intake also helps reduce caloric intake – important for control of weight and type II diabetes
- Maintain adequate dietary potassium, calcium and magnesium intake
- Relaxation techniques – biofeedback
- Vegetarian diets, fish oil

* These interventions have been found to be effective. Data on other interventions are not definitive (see text).

Modified from: JNC-V. *Arch Intern Med.* 1993;153:154-183 and JNC-VI. *Arch Intern Med.* In press.

People who exceed these limits by 20% or more are considered obese and should be started on a weight reduction program. Experience shows that liquid formulas or "crash" or "miracle" diets are ineffective over the long term. The process of losing large amounts of weight quickly leads to a downward readjustment of the metabolic rate and a gain in weight once a more normal diet is resumed. A simple, easy-to-follow weight reduction program, resulting in a loss of one or two pounds per week, is most effective. In cases

TABLE 3.2 — HOW TO ESTIMATE IDEAL BODY WEIGHT

Women — Height: 5 feet, 5 inches

Allow 100 pounds for first 5 feet of height	100
Add 5 pounds for each additional inch	+ 25
Ideal body weight for a 5-foot, 5-inch woman =	125

Men — Height: 5 feet, 10 inches

Allow 106 pounds for first 5 feet of height	106
Add 6 pounds for each additional inch	+ 60
Ideal body weight for a 5-foot, 10-inch man =	166

of morbid obesity (ie, 100% or more above ideal weight), more stringent methods should be undertaken.

In a person who usually ingests about 2,000 calories a day and is targeted to lose one pound a week, daily caloric intake should be reduced by 500 calories or, as an alternative, reduced by 300 calories and caloric expenditure increased by about 200 calories a day. An overall reduction of about 500 calories a day from the usual intake will result in a weight loss of approximately one pound a week (3,500 calories equals one pound). Table 3.3 will help a patient calculate how many calories are necessary to maintain ideal weight. This can serve as a starting point in calculating behavioral and dietary changes. Table 3.4 summarizes the caloric expenditures for various activities.

Weight loss is difficult, but if achieved and maintained, it will usually result in some decrease in blood pressure. This may be enough in some patients with slightly elevated blood pressure (Stage I) to reduce their blood pressure to normotensive levels (< 140/

TABLE 3.3 — HOW TO ESTIMATE NUMBER OF CALORIES NEEDED TO MAINTAIN IDEAL WEIGHT

Multiply ideal weight (not necessarily your present weight) by your activity level.

Ideal weight (lbs.)	125
Activity level: Sedentary .... 13 Moderately active .... 15 Very active 17	× 13
Total calories needed per day to maintain ideal weight	= 1,625

(A sedentary woman whose ideal weight is 125 will require approximately 125 × 13 or 1,625 calories/day to maintain her ideal weight.)

90 mm Hg). There is no risk and this intervention need not be costly if it is carried out without involvement in health clubs or expensive "miracle weight loss" programs.

Attempts at weight loss (if appropriate) should be begun and the patient seen again in 2 to 3 months for a repeat blood pressure check. If the blood pressure is < 140/90 mm Hg, a diagnosis of hypertension at that time is not justified; the weight loss may have been a factor in reducing pressure, but blood pressure may have come down anyway. In all of the large clinical trials, a varying percentage of people experienced a decrease in blood pressure without specific interventions. In addition to its immediate effect on blood pressure, achieving normal weight may be important in preventing diabetes or future hypertension. If, however, pressures remain elevated and specific therapy becomes

TABLE 3.4 — CALORIE EXPENDITURES FOR VARIOUS ACTIVITIES

Activity	Approximate calories burned per *half-hour*
Normal Activities	
Cleaning windows	130
Gardening	110
Mowing lawn (power mower)	125
Sitting/conversing	40
Vacuuming	130
Moderate Exercise	
Bicycling (5 mph)	105
Bicycling (8 mph)	165
Bowling	135
Playing golf (using power cart)	100
Playing golf (pulling cart)	135
Playing volleyball	175
Roller skating	175
Square dancing	175
Swimming (1/4 mph)	150
Walking (1 mph)	65
Walking (3 mph)	140
Vigorous Exercise	
Bicycling (10 mph)	195
Bicycling (13 mph)	330
Hill climbing (100 ft/hr)	245
Ice skating (10 mph)	200
Jogging (5 mph)	265
Playing squash, handball	300
Playing tennis	210
Running (8 mph)	360
Skiing (10 mph)	300
Walking (4 mph)	195

3

necessary, maintaining an ideal weight will be helpful in minimizing the amount of medication. Weight reduction of even 10 or 15 pounds (even without specific sodium restriction) will lower blood pressure in some patients.

Sodium Restriction

Conflicting reports have confused physicians about this intervention. Most people ingest more salt (sodium) than needed. The average salt intake in the United States is still approximately 10 g/day (approximately 4 g of sodium a day). Little harm would be done if every person reduced sodium intake. In a patient with even transiently elevated blood pressure, the reduction of salt intake to approximately 6 g/day (sodium to approximately 2.4 g or about 100 mmol/day) may result in a slight decrease or normalization of blood pressure. Some studies report significant decreases in blood pressure with moderate sodium restriction; others report only insignificant changes (Table 3.5). Many trials have been poorly controlled or are short term. As noted in Table 3.5, in one 8-week study (Watt) with restriction of sodium to below 60 mmol, there was no blood pressure response; yet, in a 12-month study (Silman) with a reduction of sodium excretion from 151 to just 117 mmol/day, there was a -9/-6 mm Hg reduction.

Table 3.6 lists some foods with a high sodium content. If these are avoided, many patients can reduce their sodium intake to a reasonable level and possibly lower blood pressure without further, more difficult-to-follow restrictions. More rigid salt restriction is necessary for patients with renal failure or congestive heart failure. More rigid sodium restriction (to 1 g of sodium or below 50 mmol/day) might also be effective in lowering blood pressure to a greater degree in other patients, but most people find it

TABLE 3.5 — EXAMPLES OF STUDIES OF SODIUM RESTRICTION IN HYPERTENSION TREATMENT

Study	No. of Patients	Sodium Excretion (mmol/d)		Duration	Blood Pressure (mm Hg)	
		Before	After		Baseline	Reduction
Parijs et al	22	191	93	4 wk	147/98	-7/-4
Morgan et al	28	191	157	24 wk	160/97	-2/-7
MacGregor et al	19	162	86	4 wk	156/98	-10/-5*
Beard et al	45	150	37	12 wk	142/88	-5/-3*
Watt et al	18	139	59	8 wk	150/91	—
Silman et al	12	151	117	12 mo	165/98	-9/-6

* Difference between high- and low-sodium groups.

From: Moser M. *Lower Your Blood Pressure and Live Longer.* New York, NY: Berkley Publishing Group; 1991.

TABLE 3.6 — SOME FOODS WITH A HIGH SODIUM CONTENT THAT SHOULD BE AVOIDED	
• Potato chips	• Bouillon
• Pretzels	• Ham
• Salted crackers	• Sausages
• Biscuits	• Frankfurters
• Pancakes	• Smoked meats or fish
• Fast foods	• Sardines
• Olives	• Tomato juice (canned)
• Pickles	• Frozen lima beans
• Sauerkraut	• Frozen peas
• Soy sauce	• Canned spinach
• Catsup	• Canned carrots
• Many kinds of cheese	
• Commercially prepared soups or stews	
• Pastries or cakes made from self-rising flour mixes	

From: Moser M. *Lower Your Blood Pressure and Live Longer.* New York, NY: Berkley Publishing Group; 1991.

impossible to follow this type of regimen for other than short periods.

A recent study suggesting that marked sodium restriction might actually increase the occurrence of myocardial infarction was poorly controlled. These results should not be used for treatment decisions.

Moderate salt restriction should be tried in all individuals with elevated blood pressure. There are so-called salt-sensitive subjects who will experience a definite decrease in blood pressure within a few days or weeks. In others, there may be no response at all. This individual variation in response cannot be accurately predicted. From a public health point of view, sodium restriction and weight loss or maintaining normal weight have proven to be the most effective methods for preventing hypertension.

Calcium Supplementation

Data are confusing concerning the value of calcium supplementation. Some investigators maintain the following:

- A low calcium intake predisposes patients to hypertension
- An increase in calcium intake with 1 g to 2 g of supplemental calcium lowers blood pressure

Others interpret the available data differently. Based on current data, calcium supplements cannot be recommended as effective treatment for hypertension. In postmenopausal women, supplemental calcium is probably useful in the treatment of osteoporosis.

Potassium Supplementation

A high potassium intake prevents strokes in animal models. Supplements of 60 to 100 mEq/day above the usual dietary intake of between 50 and 80 mEq/day have been shown to lower blood pressure in humans in some clinical trials. Many patients will develop gastrointestinal symptoms with this degree of potassium supplementation. A potassium intake of about 60 to 100 mEq/day is recommended regardless of whether hypertension is present. In areas like the rural South where the daily intake of potassium may be low (< 40 mEq/day) and daily intake of sodium high (> 5 g/day), there is a high prevalence of hypertension and strokes. At present, however, there is little evidence to support the use of potassium supplements as definitive therapy for hypertension. Table 3.7 lists some foods that are high in potassium.

For many years, attempts have been made to reduce sodium and increase potassium intake by the use of potassium salt substitutes. Most of these substitutes are bitter to the taste and poorly tolerated. A

TABLE 3.7 — LOW-SALT, HIGH-POTASSIUM FOODS

Food	Serving Size	Potassium* (mgs)	Sodium† (mgs)
Apricots	3 medium	281	1
Apricots (dried)	8 halves	490	13
Asparagus	6 spears	278	2
Avocado	1/2 medium	604	4
Banana	1 medium	569	1
Beans (white, cooked)	1/2 cup	416	7
Beans (green)	1 cup	189	5
Broccoli	1 stalk	267	10
Cantaloupe	1/4 medium	251	12
Carrots	2 small	341	47
Dates	10 medium	648	1
Grapefruit	1/2 medium	135	1
Mushrooms	4 large	414	15
Orange	1 medium	311	2
Orange juice	1 cup	496	3
Peach	1 medium	202	1
Peanuts (plain)	2 1/2 oz	740	2
Potato	1 medium	504	4
Prunes (dried)	8 large	940	11
Raisins	1/4 medium	271	10
Spinach	1/2 cup	291	45
Squash (acorn)	1/2 baked	749	2
Sunflower seeds	3 1/2 oz	920	30
Sweet potato	1 small	367	15
Tomato	1 small	244	3
Watermelon	1 slice (6 1/2 in)	600	6

* 1000 mg = 25.6 mmols
† 1000 mg = 44 mmols

From: Moser M. *Lower Your Blood Pressure and Live Longer*. Berkley: Putnam Books; 1992.

new substitute, Cardia Salt, which has been in use for several years in Europe, is now available in the United States. This product contains about 55% of the sodium chloride in regular salt and has added potassium and magnesium. It lacks the bitter taste of previous salt substitutes. Its use will help to increase potassium intake while at the same time reducing sodium intake.

Magnesium Supplementation

There is some evidence from animal studies that a high magnesium intake lowers blood pressure, but this has not been shown to be true in controlled studies with humans. At present, magnesium supplements cannot be recommended as a definitive method for lowering blood pressure. The JNC-V and JNC-VI recommend that an adequate intake of this mineral be maintained.

High-fiber, Low-fat Diet; Fish Oil

High-fiber, low-fat diets have also been shown to reduce blood pressure in some studies, but carefully controlled long-term studies have not been done. At present, there is little definitive evidence that this type of dietary intervention will lower blood pressure. It may, however, be effective in maintaining serum lipid levels at more desirable levels. A low-fat, high-fiber diet can therefore be recommended.

Large doses of omega-3 fatty acids may lower blood pressure to some extent, but may produce adverse reactions. A meta-analysis that included results from six trials in hypertensive patients reported a decrease of -5.5/-3.5 mm Hg in blood pressure. Dosages used were 6 to 10 capsules a day of commercially available fish oil, which are equivalent to a daily serving of 200 g of fish with a high content of omega-

3 oils (mackerel, certain kinds of salmon, etc.). This approach also cannot be recommended at this time as specific treatment for hypertension. There is no good evidence that an extra daily intake of garlic will lower blood pressure.

Alcohol Moderation

JNC-V and JNC-VI have reiterated what the previous committees recommended and numerous epidemiologic studies have reported. A low-to-moderate intake of alcohol may actually decrease cardiovascular risk, but an intake higher than 1 to 2 ounces of ethanol a day may increase blood pressure. Daily intake should not exceed 2 ounces of whiskey, 10 ounces of wine, or 24 ounces of beer. Women and thin individuals should limit their ethanol intake to approximately one half of these amounts. We have followed patients who have been diagnosed as hypertensive whose pressures have decreased to normal when alcohol intake was reduced from more than four to five drinks per day to one or none. Alcohol probably contributes to elevated blood pressure by its stimulatory effect on catecholamines. *The recommendation for a moderate intake of alcohol should obviously not be given to those with a strong family history of alcoholism or a personal sensitivity to alcohol.*

Exercise

This is another confusing issue. Several studies have found that vigorous exercise over the short term will lower blood pressure in patients with less severe hypertension, ie, between 140/90 and 160/100 mm Hg. Many of these studies were poorly controlled; in the studies that have had a control group, the difference between treated and control groups has usually not been great. On the other hand, the chance of a sedentary individual developing hypertension or a coronary event is greater than that of a physically active individual; this has been repeatedly demonstrated in long-term, prospective, epidemiologic studies.

There is some confusion over what constitutes an active person. Active does not imply involvement in vigorous aerobic exercises to achieve 75% to 80% or more of target heart rates that have been recommended by numerous physicians.

Recent data show that *cardiovascular risk* is reduced by a program involving moderate exercise. This includes walking for 30 to 40 minutes at a rate of 2 to 3 miles per hour, 3 to 4 times per week. Achieving *fitness* does require more vigorous aerobic activity, but you can be an *active* individual without being *fit*, and you may not have to achieve a high level of fitness to reduce your risk. Exercise is helpful in burning calories, thereby helping to reduce weight. Exercise may increase vasodilator hormones that lower vascular resistance and may therefore help to lower blood pressure. Exercise is recommended, but is not to be counted on as definitive antihypertensive therapy.

Relaxation Programs and Biofeedback

Numerous relaxation and biofeedback programs have been advocated for the lowering of blood pressure. These include yoga, transcendental meditation and hypnosis. Most reported studies are poorly controlled. Blood pressure may be lowered at the time someone is practicing a relaxation technique, but this should not be depended on as definitive treatment.

Table 3.8 outlines the Benson technique for relaxation. Patients can be taught to do this in a few minutes. Using this technique once or twice a day cannot hurt anyone and may periodically turn off enough adrenaline to be of some benefit. Many of our patients have found this type of relaxation to be helpful without a major time or economic commitment.

Summary of Lifestyle Changes

After the initial discovery of elevated blood pressure, the patient should be advised to:

- Reduce excess body weight by calorie restriction and exercise, if appropriate
- Reduce dietary sodium to about 6 g of sodium chloride a day (2.4 g of sodium)
- Maintain an adequate intake of potassium, calcium and magnesium without necessarily using supplements—a recently introduced low-sodium, high-potassium and magnesium salt substitute may be helpful
- Limit alcohol intake to less than 2 oz of whiskey, 10 oz of wine, or 24 oz of beer a day (approximately one half of these amounts for women and thin individuals)
- Exercise moderately within the framework of daily activity for 20 to 30 minutes, 3 to 4 times a week
- Plan some type of relaxation for short periods several times a day

In addition, because smoking and elevated lipid levels are important risk factors for heart disease, these should be corrected if present. There is no evidence that chronic smoking will cause a persistent elevation of blood pressure, but smoking may have an immediate effect on raising blood pressure, primarily because of the nicotine effect on catecholamines.

TABLE 3.8 — Dr. Herbert Benson's Relaxation Response Technique

- Sit quietly in a comfortable position.
- Close your eyes.
- Relax all your muscles, progressing from your feet to your face. Keep them relaxed.
- Breathe through your nose. As you breathe out, say the word "one" silently to yourself.
- Continue for 10 to 20 minutes. You may open your eyes to check the time, but do not set an alarm. When you finish, sit quietly for several minutes, at first with your eyes closed. Do not stand for a few minutes.
- Do not worry about achieving a deep level of relaxation. Maintain a passive attitude and permit relaxation to occur at its own pace. When distracting thoughts occur, don't dwell upon them, but return to repeating "one." With practice, the response should come with little effort. Use the technique once or twice daily, but not within 2 hours after any meal, because the digestive processes seem to interfere with elicitation of the response.

To utilize this technique once or twice a day requires an ongoing commitment of time and effort.

Adapted from: Benson H. *The Relaxation Response*. New York, NY: Times Books; 1984.

Follow-up Program

Although it may seem inappropriate to undertake any kind of intervention after only one blood pressure reading, the above rather simple nonpharmacologic interventions:

- Make good sense
- Do no harm
- Incur no cost
- Require very little time on the part of the patient.

Even if they have no effect on blood pressure, they establish a pattern of behavior that can only help to reduce the risk of heart disease.

Patients should be seen after 3 to 4 months. If blood pressure is still elevated above 140/90 mm Hg despite lifestyle interventions and the pressure is not higher than 150/95 to 150/100 mm Hg, an additional 3-month trial of nonpharmacologic intervention may be justified (although specific therapy is probably indicated if other major risk factors are present, such as smoking, diabetes or hyperlipidemia). I personally believe that specific drug therapy is a reasonable approach at this stage, even if there are no other risk factors (see Section 4, *Drug Treatment of Hypertension*). If the pressure is above 150/100 mm Hg, specific medical therapy should certainly be undertaken. On a third visit (2 to 3 months later) in subjects not already on medication, medical therapy is indicated if blood pressures are above 140/90 mm Hg. This is true whether or not left ventricular hypertrophy or any other target organ damage has been identified.

There is evidence that pharmacologic intervention in addition to lifestyle modifications at this level of blood pressure will provide beneficial effects and reduce cardiovascular risk. A study of Stage I hypertension (Treatment of Mild Hypertension Study [TOMHS]) demonstrated reduction in overall cardiovascular events after 4 years in medically treated patients whose average pretreatment blood pressures were only 140/91 mm Hg.

Some patients have been led to believe that nonpharmacologic or lifestyle interventions are all that are necessary to control their blood pressure. This is not true in most cases. The exact numbers are not known, but our experience suggests that blood pressures will be reduced to normal in fewer than 20% to 25% of all patients who have consistently elevated blood pressures and who follow the above program. We should stress that nonpharmacologic or lifestyle interventions should be continued while medications are taken, since these interventions may help to reduce pressures somewhat further and have been shown to augment the effects of medication.

Long-term outcome may be adversely effected if lifestyle modifications are continued without medication, despite persistently elevated blood pressures.

3

4

Drug Treatment of Hypertension: General Information

Opinions differ as to when medication should be started. Patients with blood pressures in the range of about 140/90 to 150/100 mm Hg are usually in no immediate danger of a cardiovascular event, and drug therapy can be postponed while lifestyle modification is given a chance to work. As noted, blood pressures may decrease on repeated observations. This may be secondary to:

- Lifestyle interventions
- Acclimatization to the blood pressure cuff
- A result of the "regression to the mean" phenomenon (in large groups, people at the extremes tend to gravitate to the mean or average).

There is good evidence, however, to suggest that if blood pressures remain above 140/90 mm Hg after 3 to 6 months of lifestyle intervention (as outlined in Section 3, *Lifestyle Modifications*), medication is indicated.

Some physicians continue to advocate lifestyle management without specific medication unless the diastolic pressures are consistently above 95 to 100 mm Hg or unless other definite risk factors are present such as:

- Diabetes
- Obesity
- Hyperlipidemia.

It is well established that at least the short-term benefit of treatment is greatest in higher risk individuals, ie, the elderly, persons with the highest blood pressures, or those with additional risk factors. For this reason, the JNC-VI advocates more immediate therapy in these subjects, but some delay in patients with lower pressures and no other risk factors. For example, in a person under the age of 60 with Stage I hypertension (blood pressures between 140-159/90-99 mm Hg) and no other risk factors, lifestyle modifications might be continued for 9 to 12 months. However, if left ventricular hypertrophy (LVH) or diabetes is present, specific medical therapy in addition to lifestyle changes might be started as soon as the diagnosis is made.

While I agree with this concept, physicians might be cautioned not to delay medications too long. We should not forget the lessons from the 1930s and 1940s when all we had to offer the patient with hypertension were low-sodium diets, weight loss, phenobarbital or mutilating surgery, such as a sympathectomy. In the days before effective therapy became available, so-called mild hypertension frequently progressed to malignant or accelerated hypertension, congestive heart failure, strokes and other complications of hypertension. These phenomena are rare today in well-treated patients. The risk for cerebrovascular and cardiovascular complications are decreased with effective blood pressure lowering. A suggested approach to specific initial therapy is outlined in Table 4.1.

Beneficial Effects of Long-term Therapy

A recent meta-analysis of 3- to 5-year clinical trials, including trials in the elderly, shows a highly statistically significant decrease in stroke deaths (40%) and coronary disease deaths (16%) compared with

TABLE 4.1 — SUGGESTED APPROACH TO MANAGEMENT OF A PATIENT WITH INITIAL BLOOD PRESSURE ≥ 140/90 MM HG*

BP 140/90 – 150/100 MM HG

Lifestyle interventions for 2 to 3 or up to 6 months, depending on age and presence or absence of other risk factors:
- Weight loss if appropriate†
- Sodium restriction to 2 to 2.5 g/day†
- Exercise program (moderate and repetitive)
- Adequate intake of potassium, calcium and magnesium
- Limit alcohol intake to less than 2 oz whiskey, 10 oz wine, 24 oz beer (approximately one half of these amounts for women and thin individuals)
- Smoking cessation; low-fat, high-fiber diet
- Practice some form of relaxation technique.

After this period of initial observation, there are several options:‡

A. **BP < 140/90 mm Hg:**
   Continue above—see patient in 6 months

B. **BP 140/90–150/100 mm Hg:**
   Continue above—*probably begin drug therapy*

BP > 150/100-105 mm Hg

Specific drug therapy PLUS lifestyle interventions
If after 1 year blood pressure has remained within normal limits, medication can be withdrawn gradually to see if normotensive levels are maintained by nonpharmacologic means.

---

* Three readings taken a few minutes apart in the sitting position.
† Most effective nonpharmacologic interventions.
‡ See text for detailed information.

control groups or placebo (Figure 4.1). These trials achieved an average decrease of only 5 to 6 mm Hg diastolic and approximately 10 to 12 mm Hg systolic in treated groups compared with either placebo or control groups. Approximately 25% to 30% of patients did not even reach goal pressures, and in some instances, goal pressures were set as high as 95 mm Hg diastolic. Even better results might have been expected if a higher percentage of patients had been treated to a goal of below 90 mm Hg diastolic. These recent data have clearly invalidated the argument that coronary heart disease (CHD) events are not decreased by long-term lowering of blood pressure.

In addition to a reduction in strokes, stroke deaths and overall cardiovascular deaths, treatment has:

- Prevented progression from less severe to more severe disease, a factor not often considered when the trials are analyzed (only 95 of 13,389 persons in treated groups compared with 1,493 of 13,342 in the placebo or control groups progressed to severe hypertension [defined as diastolic pressure of 110 to 130 mm Hg or higher and/or a systolic pressure of 210 to 230 mm Hg or higher]) (see Section 16, *Results of Therapy*)
- Reduced congestive heart failure (CHF) as a complication of hypertension by more than 50%—in the 1940s, CHF accounted for about 40% of the deaths in hypertensive patients. Hypertensive heart disease was the most common cause of CHF; and
- Prevented LVH or caused a regression of LVH in a large number of patients following the lowering of blood pressure (see Section 16, *Results of Therapy*).

There are, therefore, sufficient data to justify the treatment of hypertensive patients, even those with Stage I hypertension and no evidence of target organ involvement. Management should stress:

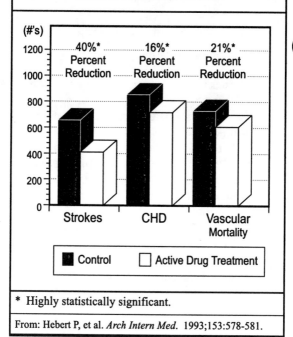

FIGURE 4.1 — EFFECT OF ANTIHYPERTENSIVE DRUG TREATMENT ON CORONARY HEART DISEASE, STROKES AND VASCULAR MORTALITY IN SEVENTEEN 3- TO 5-YEAR CLINICAL TRIALS

* Highly statistically significant.

From: Hebert P, et al. *Arch Intern Med.* 1993;153:578-581.

- Keeping the treatment as uncomplicated as possible
- Keeping dosages of medication low to minimize side effects
- Making all efforts to increase adherence to a therapy regimen.

In our experience, fewer than 10% of patients will discontinue medication because of side effects if the medications are chosen carefully and dosages kept at the lower part of the recommended range. Some studies suggest that as many as 30% to 40% of patients discontinue therapy because of side effects, but this has not been our experience.

Factors Influencing Outcome of Therapy

Several factors determine the success of medical therapy:

- Physicians should choose a drug proven to be effective in a high percentage of patients. In our experience, a higher percentage of patients will achieve normotensive levels if a diuretic rather than another drug is used as initial therapy, especially in Black subjects or in subjects over 50 to 55 years of age. Recent trials suggest, however, that any one of the drugs in five of the six classes currently suggested as first-step or alternative initial therapy will lower blood pressure to an *almost* equivalent degree (diuretics, β-blockers, ACE inhibitors, calcium channel blockers [CCBs], α_1-blockers) (Table 4.2).

- Blood pressure should be titrated to goal levels. Too many patients with pressures of 160/100 mm Hg, for example, are inadequately treated. Blood pressures decrease to 145-150/90-95 mm Hg and medication is not changed. If the full benefit of therapy is to be achieved, blood pressures should be decreased to < 140/90 mm Hg, if possible. In our experience, more than 80% of patients achieve goal pressures with a simple, relatively inexpensive regimen. This frequently requires small doses of different classes of medications (eg, a diuretic plus an ACE inhibitor or β-blocker). Patients are seen only 2, or at most 3, times a year once

TABLE 4.2 — AVERAGE BLOOD PRESSURE (BP) CHANGE FROM BASELINE AT 48 MONTHS FOR PATIENTS IN THE TREATMENT OF MILD HYPERTENSION STUDY (TOMHS)*

	Treatment Groups					
NO—	Acebutolol	Amlodipine	Chlorthalidone	Doxazosin	Enalapril	Placebo[†]
	126	114	117	121	119	207
Systolic BP, mm Hg change at 48 months	-13.9	-14.1	-14.6	-13.4	-11.3	-8.6
Diastolic BP, mm Hg change at 48 months	-11.5	-12.2	-11.1	-11.2	-9.7	-8.6

* Baseline average BP was 140/91 mm Hg. Nutritional intervention (placebo cohort) resulted in a decrease of 8.6/8.6 mm Hg in BP. Medication, in addition to lifestyle changes, resulted in an additional decrease of about 5 mm Hg systolic (except with enalapril) and about 3 mm Hg diastolic (except for enalapril). These slight additional decreases in BP resulted in an overall decrease in cardiovascular morbidity and mortality.

† Nutritional intervention only.

From: Neaton JD, et al. *JAMA*. 1993;270:713-724.

blood pressure control is achieved. This may suggest patient neglect, but good results have also been achieved in the major clinical trials (eg, the Hypertension Detection and Follow-up Program) where patients were seen only 3 to 4 times a year. Follow-up visits during the first 6 months of therapy may have to be more frequent to achieve blood pressure control.

- Patient education is important in gaining cooperation and helping patients to understand the reasons for therapy. We have used a booklet entitled *High Blood Pressure and What You Can Do About It* for many years to help in this effort. It is available free from the National Center for Health Information, 120/80; P.O. Box 30105; Bethesda, MD 20824-0015. In addition, a paperback book, *Lower Your Blood Pressure and Live Longer* (Avon Books), is available and should be helpful to patients in explaining the management of hypertension. Occasionally, home blood pressure recording is helpful in demonstrating to the patient that blood pressures have been lowered. Home blood pressure can be determined with one of the many inexpensive ($25 to $50) sphygmomanometers on the market; ambulatory blood pressure monitoring is rarely necessary.

- Keep the cost of therapy as low as possible. As many as 20% to 25% of people are unable to afford to fill their prescriptions. In addition, many become discouraged with the process of treatment when expensive diagnostic testing is used (see Section 2, *Diagnosis*).

The So-called J-shaped Curve

There is little evidence from an analysis of the clinical trials that reducing blood pressure below a certain level increases CHD risk. Some investigators, however, believe that CHD events actually increase if diastolic blood pressures are reduced below 80 to 85 mm Hg. This conclusion is based on small numbers of patients and extrapolation from larger sets of data. But in the Systolic Hypertension in the Elderly Program (SHEP), for example, where diastolic blood pressures were reduced to below 70 mm Hg, patients showed a decrease, not an increase, in CHD mortality. At present, there is little evidence to suggest that there is a limit below which blood pressure should not be reduced. Long-term studies are presently underway to define this issue.

Specific Drug Therapy

The Sixth Report of the Joint National Committee on Detection, Evaluation and Treatment of High Blood Pressure (JNC-VI) published in 1997 represents the opinions of nine executive committee members and approximately 100 consultants. The Report has been approved by most medical organizations involved in the diagnosis and treatment of hypertension in the United States. After reviewing the available data, the Committee concluded that "when the decision has been made to begin antihypertensive therapy and if there are no indications for another type of drug, a diuretic or β-blocker should be chosen." This recommendation was based on evidence from the long-term clinical trials which used these agents and found a significant reduction in not only cerebrovascular but cardiovascular morbidity and mortality in treated compared to control or placebo patients. This specific recommendation is similar to that of the JNC-V.

The JNC-VI specifically designated special situations for the use of the following drugs (see Section 15, *Approach to Therapy* and Tables 15.1 and 15.2 for details):

- ACE inhibitors
- Angiotensin II receptor antagonists
- CCBs
- α_1–β-Blockers
- α-Blockers.

In addition, the committee suggested that fixed-dose combinations (ie, a diuretic/β-blocker, diuretic/ACE inhibitor, diuretic/angiotensin II receptor antagonist, ACE inhibitor/CCB) might be appropriate initial therapy.

The new recommendations also suggest that there may be more compelling reasons to use various medications in certain situations. For example, if a physician sees a patient with heart failure who is not receiving an ACE inhibitor and a diuretic, these agents should be added. Similarly, if a diuretic is not being used in the treatment of isolated systolic hypertension (ISH), it should be substituted or added to therapy. A CCB may be used if a diuretic is contraindicated or not effective. In myocardial infarction patients, there is a strong reason to use a non-ISA β-blocker. In subjects with systolic dysfunction, an ACE inhibitor or angiotensin II receptor antagonist is indicated.

It is possible that when studies presently under way are concluded, ACE inhibitors, angiotensin II receptor antagonists and possibly at least some of the CCBs will prove to be as effective in reducing morbidity and mortality as those agents that have been tested to date. There are indications from several short-term trials that medications which interfere with the renin-angiotensin system (ie, ACE inhibitors or angiotensin II receptor antagonists) will prove effective in long-term trials, especially if they are used with a diuretic. At present, however, there is no definitive proof of this. One recently reported randomized, controlled study (Syst Eur) with a long-acting dihydropyrimidine CCB, nitrendipine (not available in the United States), has demonstrated a reduction in fatal and nonfatal strokes and a trend toward reduction of cardiovascular events in elderly subjects primarily with ISH.

Figure 4.2 represents our modification of the JNC-VI recommendations. We favor the use of small doses of two different classes of drugs if monotherapy is ineffective, rather than sequential monotherapy (see Section 15, *Approach to Therapy*, for details), unless blood pressure is not lowered at all by the first agent chosen or troublesome side effects occur.

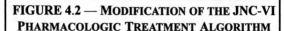

FIGURE 4.2 — MODIFICATION OF THE JNC-VI PHARMACOLOGIC TREATMENT ALGORITHM

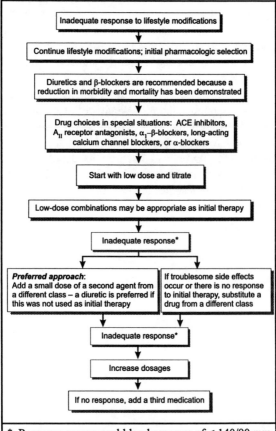

Inadequate response to lifestyle modifications

Continue lifestyle modifications; initial pharmacologic selection

Diuretics and β-blockers are recommended because a reduction in morbidity and mortality has been demonstrated

Drug choices in special situations: ACE inhibitors, A_{II} receptor antagonists, α_1–β-blockers, long-acting calcium channel blockers, or α-blockers

Start with low dose and titrate

Low-dose combinations may be appropriate as initial therapy

Inadequate response*

Preferred approach:
Add a small dose of a second agent from a different class – a diuretic is preferred if this was not used as initial therapy

If troublesome side effects occur or there is no response to initial therapy, substitute a drug from a different class

Inadequate response*

Increase dosages

If no response, add a third medication

* Response means goal blood pressure of < 140/90 mm Hg has been achieved or patient is making considerable progress toward this goal.

Modified from: JNC-VI. *Arch Intern Med.* In press.

5 Diuretics

Diuretics have been used successfully since the middle 1950s in the management of hypertension. Table 5.1 lists the most commonly used diuretics in the United States. (*Tables in this section may not include all of the available preparations in each class of drugs*; for a more complete list, see the Sixth Report of the Joint National Committee on Detection, Evaluation and Treatment of High Blood Pressure [JNC-VI. *Arch Intern Med*. In press].) The duration of action varies considerably among the various thiazide derivatives and other orally effective agents.

Diuretics can be divided into several classes:

- *Thiazide or thiazide-type diuretics,* which block the reabsorption of sodium in the early distal tubule
- *Indoline derivatives*
- *Loop diuretics,* which act more proximally and block sodium reabsorption in the loop of Henle—these are more potent in terms of their natriuretic effect since they act on the glomerular filtrate early in the nephron
- *Potassium-sparing diuretics,* which act in the distal tubule, thereby preventing some of the exchange of sodium for potassium that occurs in this portion of the nephron (Figure 5.1).

The longer-acting thiazide diuretics are more effective as antihypertensive drugs than the loop diuretics in the dosages that are usually administered. The most commonly used thiazide diuretics in the United States are the following:

- Hydrochlorothiazide, with a duration of action of approximately 12 to 18 hours

TABLE 5.1 — SOME COMMONLY USED DIURETICS FOR TREATING HYPERTENSION

Diuretic Generic (Trade) Name	Recommended Dosage Range		Duration of Action (Hours)	Comments
	Dose (mg)	Frequency		
Thiazide and Related Agents				
Chlorthalidone (Hygroton)	12.5-50	1/day	24-72	More effective than loop diuretics except in patients with serum creatinine > 2.5 mg/dL—hydrochlorothiazide and chlorthalidone were used in most clinical trials
Hydrochlorothiazide (Esidrix, Hydrodiuril, Microzide)	12.5-50	1-2/day	12-18	
Methyclothiazide (Enduron)	2.5-5	1/day	> 24	
Metolazone (Diulo, Mykrox, Zaroxolyn)	0.5-5	1/day	18-24	A relatively low-sodium and high-potassium diet may help to augment BP lowering and prevent hypokalemia
Indoline Derivatives				
Indapamide (Lozol)	1.25-5	1/day	18-24	

Loop Diuretics			
Bumetanide (Bumex)	0.5-4	2/day	4-6	Not usually used as initial therapy in hypertension. Higher doses may be needed for patients with renal impairment or congestive heart failure — ethacrynic acid is only alternative for patients with allergy to sulfur-containing diuretics
Ethacrynic acid (Edecrin)	25-100	2-3/day	6-8	
Furosemide (Lasix)	20-320	2-3/day	6-8	
Torsemide (Demadex)	2.5-20	1/day*	6-12+	Long duration of action may make this more suitable for treatment of hypertensive patients
Potassium-sparing Diuretics			
Amiloride (Midamor) as part of Moduretic	5-10	1 or 2/day	18-24	Weak diuretics—used mainly in combination with other diuretics to avoid or reverse hypokalemia; avoid when serum creatinine > 2.5 mg/dL or in patients receiving an ACE inhibitor; may cause hyperkalemia
Triamterene (Dyrenium) as part of Dyazide or Maxzide	25-150	1 or 2/day	7-9	
Spironolactone (Aldactone) as part of Aldactazide	25-100	2 or 3/day	8-12	

* Effect on blood pressure is longer than other loop diuretics.

55

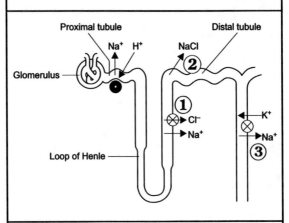

FIGURE 5.1 — SITE OF ACTION OF DIURETICS

Key: ①, loop diuretics; ②, thiazides; ③, potassium-sparing agents.

- Chlorthalidone, with a duration of action of more than 24 hours
- An indoline derivative, indapamide, with a duration of action of about 18 to 24 hours.

Potassium-sparing diuretics are usually not used by themselves; they are weak diuretics and are relatively ineffective in lowering blood pressure when used alone. Various combinations of thiazides and potassium-sparing agents are available (eg, Dyazide, Maxzide, Moduretic, Aldactazide).

Mechanism of Action

The exact mechanism of action of diuretics in lowering blood pressure is not known, although they have been used for 40 years. Initially, there is a decrease in plasma volume with a lowering of blood pressure and a short-term decrease in cardiac output. Over time, however:

- Cardiac output returns to normal levels
- Blood pressure remains low
- Plasma volume returns to just slightly below pretreatment levels
- Vascular resistance decreases.

The decrease in resistance is noticed both before and after exercise. Diuretics, in effect, act as vasodilators. With a persistent reduction of plasma volume, however, the renin-angiotensin-aldosterone system continues to be stimulated (Figure 5.2). This effect is not usually great enough to negate diuretic-induced vasodilation and blood pressure reduction. Figure 5.3 summarizes these actions.

Approximately 50% to 60% of patients will respond to diuretics even when given in relatively small doses. As with many antihypertensive agents, the dose-response curve of diuretics is relatively flat. A dose of 12.5 mg of hydrochlorothiazide or its equivalent will reduce blood pressure in approximately one-half to two-thirds of patients who are responsive to this class of medication. Increasing the dose to 25 mg will add another 10% to 15% to the responders. At 50 mg of hydrochlorothiazide or its equivalent, probably 80% to 90% of possible responders will have experienced a blood pressure decrease. A dose of 100 mg may add a few patients to the response list or decrease the blood pressure to a slightly greater extent, but probably at the cost of additional side effects. This is why we believe that it is more appropriate to give a small or moderate dose of a diuretic; if this does not achieve normotensive levels of blood pressure, the physician should add a small dose of another drug from another class (eg, ACE inhibitor, angiotensin II receptor antagonist or β-blocker) that might block or interfere with some of the homeostatic mechanisms

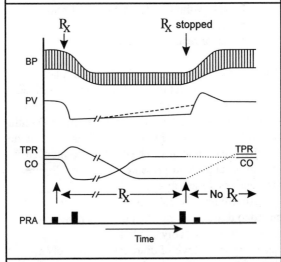

FIGURE 5.2 — HEMODYNAMIC EFFECTS OF CHLOROTHIAZIDE IN A HYPERTENSIVE PATIENT

Abbreviations: R_x, drug therapy; BP, blood pressure; PV, plasma volume; TPR, total peripheral resistance; CO, cardiac output; PRA, plasma-renin activity.

After about 4 to 6 weeks of treatment, BP remains below pretreatment levels, cardiac output has returned to normal, and vascular resistance is reduced, but plasma volume remains slightly below pretreatment levels. Resistance and BP return to pretreatment levels when diuretic is stopped.

From: Tarazi RC, et al. *Circulation*. 1970;41:709-717.

activated by the drug's effect on the renin-angiotensin-aldosterone system. We prefer this approach to therapy with small doses of different agents, regardless of which medication is used initially. A more complete review of therapy will be outlined in Section 15, *Approach to Therapy*.

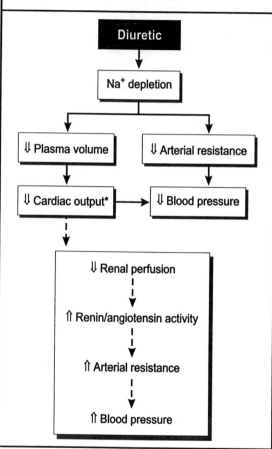

FIGURE 5.3 — PHYSIOLOGIC EFFECTS OF DIURETICS

Diuretic

↓

Na⁺ depletion

↓ Plasma volume   ↓ Arterial resistance

↓ Cardiac output* → ↓ Blood pressure

↓ Renal perfusion

↓

⇑ Renin/angiotensin activity

↓

⇑ Arterial resistance

↓

⇑ Blood pressure

* Returns to normal after several weeks.

The ultimate result of diuretic therapy is reduction of arterial resistance and blood pressure. However, a continuing increase in the activity of the renin-angiotensin system is noted. This does not, in most cases, negate the BP response, but can be counteracted in nonresponsive patients by the addition of small doses of an ACE inhibitor, a β-blocker, or an angiotensin II receptor antagonist.

Studies have shown that diuretics decrease blood pressure by approximately 10-15/5-10 mm Hg more than placebo.

Side Effects

Diuretics are as well tolerated as any of the other antihypertensive drugs. In the Veterans Administration and the Treatment of Mild Hypertension Studies (TOMHS), only about 3% of patients on these agents withdrew because of side effects. This is the lowest percentage of any of the other five classes of drugs tested against placebo. The most annoying side effect of diuretic therapy is sexual dysfunction, which, in our experience, occurs in about 5% to 10% of patients. This occurs most frequently in men, but can also be seen in women in the form of decreased libido and delay in orgasm. It can sometimes be attenuated by:

- Decreasing the dosage
- Using therapy on alternate days
- Omitting the drug for 2 or 3 days at a time.

Sexual dysfunction may cease to be a problem when the diuretic is stopped. Since this problem often occurs in men who are 60 years of age and older, however, there may not be an improvement in impotence or loss of libido (ie, medication may have had nothing to do with the dysfunction). Data from the Treatment of Mild Hypertension Study (TOMHS) suggests that a high percentage of hypertensive patients have some sexual dysfunction prior to specific therapy.

Skin rashes or photosensitivity are rare; pancreatitis is extremely rare, but can occur. In men with symptomatic prostatic hypertrophy, symptoms may be worsened.

The significance of the metabolic changes that may occur with the use of diuretics has been debated for many years (Table 5.2). In our opinion, the negative aspects of these have been overstated. It is important to clarify this issue.

■ Hypokalemia

About 30% of patients will experience a decrease in serum potassium of about 0.5 to 0.8 mEq/L on doses of 50 to 100 mg/day of hydrochlorothiazide or its equivalent. This change is dose related; on lower doses of 25 mg, the decrease is usually less than 0.3 to 0.4 mEq/L. Reports that diuretic-induced hypokalemia resulted in increased ectopy, ventricular tachycardia or sudden death have not been confirmed by recent 24- and 48-hour Holter monitor studies. These have shown that, despite the occurrence of hypokalemia, there is little increase in single ventricular premature beats, couplets or episodes of ventricular tachycardia (Table 5.3). Hypokalemia should be avoided, however, if possible, especially in:

- The elderly
- Patients on digitalis
- Patients with diabetes where the degree of hypokalemia may affect insulin utilization.

We therefore almost invariably use a potassium-sparing thiazide combination as initial therapy in these patients. This does not add significantly to the cost and eliminates the need for potassium supplements or careful monitoring. Normokalemia is not, however, achieved in all cases, especially if high doses of the diuretic are used. Many of the available thiazide- and potassium-sparing combination agents actually contain a small amount of the thiazide component (12.5 mg to a maximum of 50 mg or the equivalent of hydrochlorothiazide [HCTZ]). Blood pressure lowering is maintained, and metabolic changes are mini-

TABLE 5.2 — POTENTIAL METABOLIC CHANGES WITH DIURETIC USE

Metabolic Change	Comments
Hypokalemia	Less marked with lower dosages; avoid if possible, especially in diabetics and patients receiving digitalis
Hyperlipidemia	*Short term*—an increase of 5% to 7% in total cholesterol and low density lipoproteins (may be less with smaller dose); no effect on high density lipoproteins. *Long term—little effect*
Increased insulin resistance	Insulin resistance increased, but only slight increase in blood glucose levels in long-term trials in diuretic-treated compared with placebo subjects, no difference in new-onset diabetes when compared with other medications. Overall cardiovascular mortality reduced to same degree in diabetics as in nondiabetics
Hyperuricemia	Gout in about 3% to 5% of patients; if diuretic essential in management, allopurinol can be given
Hypercalcemia	May be advantage in treatment of osteoporosis and prevention of fractures

TABLE 5.3 — VENTRICULAR ECTOPY IN PATIENTS WITH OR WITHOUT LEFT VENTRICULAR HYPERTROPHY BEFORE AND AFTER HYDROCHLOROTHIAZIDE* (50 TO 100 MG/DAY FOR 4 WEEKS)

	LVH (n = 28)		No LVH (n = 16)	
	Baseline	Diuretic	Baseline	Diuretic
LVPWT	1.39	—	1.03	—
PK (mEq/L)	4.06	3.39	4.10	3.33
PVC/h	16.6	10.1	2.1	3.0
Total couplets	123.0	15.0	6.0	3.0
Total VT episodes	5.0	3.0	2.0	0.0

Abbreviations: LVH, left ventricular hypertrophy; LVPWT, left ventricular posterior wall thickness; PK, plasma potassium; PVC, premature ventricular contractions; VT, ventricular tachycardia.

* No increase in ectopy following high-dose diuretic therapy in subjects with or without LVH.

From: Papademetriou V, et al. *Arch Intern Med.* 1988;148:1272.

mized. *In the dosages now recommended for most of the orally effective diuretics, low potassium levels are not usually a problem.* In fixed-dose combinations with β-blockers, ACE inhibitors and angiotensin II receptor antagonists, dosages of 6.25 mg or 12.5 mg of HCTZ greatly increase the blood pressure lowering effects of the other agents with essentially no metabolic effects.

■ Effects on Lipids

Thiazide diuretics may increase cholesterol levels by about 5% to 7% within the first 3 to 12 months of therapy. The effect on high density lipoproteins (HDL) cholesterol is minimal or nonexistent; low density lipoprotein (LDL) increases parallel the effect on total cholesterol. However, in the 3- to 5-year clinical trials, there is little or no change in cholesterol levels following the use of even high-dose diuretic therapy (Table 5.4). In most of the studies, there was actually a decrease in cholesterol levels over time, especially in those patients with hyperlipidemia; this change may be secondary to "regression to the mean." For example, in the Hypertension Detection and Follow-up Program (HDFP), cholesterol levels in patients who entered the study with levels of 280 mg/dL or above decreased, those at levels of 200 mg/dL increased slightly; and levels of patients in the 220 to 230 mg/dL remained the same over a 5-year period (Figure 5.4). Thus, there is little evidence that diuretics should be avoided in patients with hyperlipidemia if these medications are necessary to lower blood pressure. As noted, there is also little evidence to suggest that any short-term effect on lipids counteracts the beneficial effects of the lowering of blood pressure—coronary heart disease events have been decreased to a statistically significant degree in diuretic-based therapy programs.

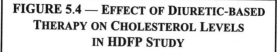

FIGURE 5.4 — EFFECT OF DIURETIC-BASED THERAPY ON CHOLESTEROL LEVELS IN HDFP STUDY

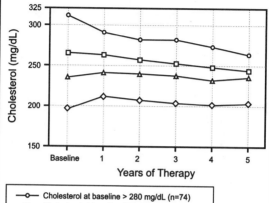

Subjects with pretreatment levels > 280 mg/dL experienced a decrease (see text).

From: Hypertension Detection and Follow-up Program Cooperative Group. *JAMA*. 1979;242:2562.

In the Systolic Hypertension in the Elderly (SHEP) and Hypertension Detection and Follow-up Program (HDFP) studies, both of which were diuretic based, morbidity and mortality for cardiovascular diseases were reduced to the same degree in patients with low and high serum cholesterol levels.

■ Insulin Resistance

Some data indicate that insulin resistance is increased in diuretic-treated patients, whereas, with some other therapies, such as ACE inhibitors, insulin

TABLE 5.4 — EFFECT OF DIURETIC-BASED THERAPY ON SERUM CHOLESTEROL IN LONG-TERM CLINICAL TRIALS*

| Trial | Duration | Total cholesterol level (mg/dL) | | Difference |
		Baseline	Medication	
Berglund & Anderson	6 yrs	267	255	-12
MRC Trial: Men/Women — active treatment — placebo	3+ yrs	245/261 244/260	245/260 239/256	0/-1 -5/-4
MAPHY	6 yrs	244	243	-1
HDFP [SC [stepped-care] group); relatively high doses of diuretics	4 yrs	232	223	-9
Oslo — active treatment — control	4 yrs	272 278	273 280	+1 +2
MRFIT — SI (special intervention) group — UC (usual care) group	6 yrs	254 254	236 240	-18 -14
HAPPHY Trial	4 yrs	242	242	—

EWPHE	— active treatment	3 yrs	256	238	-18
	— placebo		259	239	-20
MRC in Elderly	— active treatment	5 yrs	228	232	+4
	— placebo		228	232	+4
Jeunemâtre, et al		20 mos	228	232	+4
SHEP		5 yrs	—	—	2.2†
TOMHS	— active treatment	2 yrs	231	226.5	-4.5
	— placebo		225	219.9	-5.1
VA Multi-drug		2 yrs	‡	—	—

Abbreviations: MRC, Medical Research Council Study; MAPHY, Metoprolol Atherosclerosis Prevention in Hypertension Study; HDFP, Hypertension Detection and Follow-up Program; MRFIT, Multiple Risk Factor Intervention Trial; HAPPHY, Heart Attack Primary Prevention in Hypertension; EWPHE, European Working Party on High Blood Pressure in the Elderly; SHEP, Systolic Hypertension in the Elderly Program; TOMHS, Treatment of Mild Hypertension Study; VA, Veterans Administration.

* Most of the trials used diuretics in doses equivalent to 50 mg or more per day of hydrochlorothiazide.
† 2.2% more in diuretic group vs. placebo developed cholesterol levels > 300 mg/dL *at any time.*
‡ No significant differences in any lipid fractions among six classes of drugs (including diuretics) and placebo at 1 and 2 years of treatment.

From: Moser M. *Cleve Clin J Med.* 1993;60:27-37.

resistance may not change or may actually improve (Table 5.5). The clinical significance of this finding awaits further clarification. Serum glucose levels in the 3- to 5-year clinical trials were increased to only a slight degree (Table 5.6), and there was only a minimal increase in the incidence of new-onset diabetes (admittedly, none of the trials were designed to look specifically at this issue). As noted, these trials were diuretic-based, but also used other agents such as β-blockers or centrally acting agents to lower blood pressure.

One could argue that since insulin resistance is increased in many hypertensive patients before therapy, any medication that might make this worse should be avoided. It should have been expected that in a group of middle-aged or older patients with pre-treatment abnormalities in insulin resistance who were exposed to a medication that had a significant effect on glucose metabolism, diabetes would have occurred in a reasonable percentage, even over the relatively short 3- to 5-year time period of the trials. This was not noted.

Data have also demonstrated that:

- Diabetics treated with diuretics experienced a greater decrease in coronary heart disease events and mortality than nondiabetics (Figure 5.5).
- In a follow-up of a large number of hypertensive patients, those treated with diuretics did not go on to require antidiabetic therapy any more frequently than did patients treated with ACE inhibitors, β-adrenergic inhibitors, calcium channel blockers (CCBs) or α-blockers (Figure 5.6). Thus, there is little evidence that patients with diabetes or with a potential for diabetes should not be treated with diuretics if these agents are necessary to lower blood pressure.

TABLE 5.5 — CHANGES IN BLOOD GLUCOSE AND INSULIN LEVELS FOLLOWING USE OF A DIURETIC OR ACE INHIBITOR*

Variable	Study Group	Placebo (Week 0)	End of Week 18	P_1[†]	P_2[‡]
Fasting plasma Glucose (mmol/L)	C	5.7	5.5	NS	} < 0.01
	H	5.3	5.9	< 0.001	
Fasting plasma Insulin (pmol/L)	C	64	60	NS	} < 0.05
	H	54	71	< 0.01	

Abbreviations: C, captopril; H, hydrochlorothiazide; NS, not significant.

* Four-month study demonstrating an increase in insulin levels (- insulin resistance) and glucose levels in diuretic treatment compared to ACE inhibition treatment subjects.

† P_1 = difference between the effects of treatment and placebo.

‡ P_2 = difference between treatments.

From: Pollare T, et al. *N Engl J Med.* 1989;321:868.

5

TABLE 5.6 — EFFECTS OF HIGH-DOSE DIURETIC THERAPY ON GLUCOSE METABOLISM			
Study	Duration/Years	Serum Glucose (mg/dL)	Hyperglycemia or Diabetes
Oslo	5	No difference—diuretics; placebo	No specific data available
EWPHE	3	Increase 6.6—diuretics; placebo	Excess of 6/1000 patient years
MRC	3	No specific data available	Excess of 6/1000 patient years
HAPPHY	4	No specific data available	Excess of 6/1000 patient years
HDFP	5	No specific data available	1.6% (57/3563)
SHEP	1	Difference of 5 mg/dL—diuretics; placebo	1 of 483
	5	Not reported	Excess of 2.0% developed glucose levels > 200 mg/dL *at any time* in treated groups in 5 years compared with placebo

MRFIT	6	No specific data available	Excess of 7%—special intervention group with diuretics vs. excess of 2%—usual care group without diuretics*
VA	2	Increase of 1.7—diuretics; placebo	No specific data available
TOMHS	1	Decrease of 0.9—diuretics Decrease of 3.2—placebo	No specific data available

Abbreviations: EWPHE, European Working Party on High Blood Pressure in the Elderly; MRC, Medical Research Council Study; HAPPHY, Heart Attack Primary Prevention in Hypertension; HDFP, Hypertension Detection and Follow-up Program; SHEP, Systolic Hypertension in the Elderly Program; MRFIT, Multiple Risk Factor Intervention Trial; VA, Veterans Administration single-drug therapy for hypertension in men; TOMHS, Treatment of Mild Hypertension Study.

* Fasting glucose ≥ 110 mg/dL.

From: Moser M. *Cleve Clin J Med.* 1993;60:27-37.

FIGURE 5.5 — REDUCTION IN MORBIDITY AND MORTALITY IN DIABETIC* AND NONDIABETIC[†] SUBJECTS IN THE SHEP STUDY[‡]

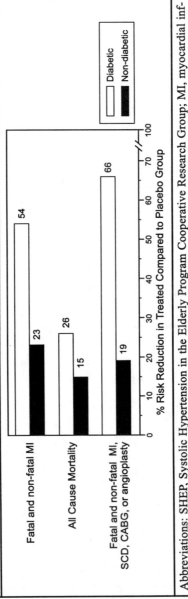

% Risk Reduction in Treated Compared to Placebo Group

Legend:
- ☐ Diabetic
- ■ Non-diabetic

Categories:
- Fatal and non-fatal MI — 54 (Diabetic), 23 (Non-diabetic)
- All Cause Mortality — 26 (Diabetic), 15 (Non-diabetic)
- Fatal and non-fatal MI, SCD, CABG, or angioplasty — 66 (Diabetic), 19 (Non-diabetic)

Abbreviations: SHEP, Systolic Hypertension in the Elderly Program Cooperative Research Group; MI, myocardial infarction; SCD, sudden cardiac death; CABG, coronary artery bypass surgery.

* Therapy group = 283 subjects, placebo group = 300 subjects.
† Therapy group = 2,080 subjects, placebo group = 2,069 subjects.
‡ Low-dose diuretic as initial therapy; β-blocker added if necessary.

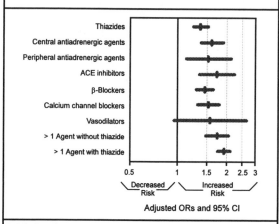

FIGURE 5.6 — RISK OF HYPERGLYCEMIA WITH USE OF ANTIHYPERTENSIVE DRUGS

Risk for development of hyperglycemia requiring treatment with antidiabetic drugs in users of antihypertensive drugs relative to nonusers (no difference between drugs).

From: Gurwitz GH, et al. *Ann Intern Med.* 1993;118:273-278.

Both serum lipids and blood glucose levels should be checked approximately 3 to 6 months after initiating therapy to detect those few patients who may experience some significant changes in these metabolic parameters. If such a change is noted, a more careful follow-up may be necessary. This extra blood test will not add significantly to treatment cost and represents good medical care in the treatment of a hypertensive individual, regardless of the medication used.

■ **Hyperuricemia**

Thiazide diuretics increase serum uric acid levels by about 0.8 to 1.5 mg % and precipitate gouty attacks, especially in susceptible individuals, in about 3% to 5% of patients. The effect on uric acid is attenuated with the smaller doses that are now used, compared with those previously recommended in the 1980s. With dosages currently suggested as initial therapy by the JNC-VI (approximately 12.5 or 25 mg of hydrochlorothiazide, 12.5 mg of chlorthalidone, 1.25 to 2.5 mg of indapamide, etc.), the incidence of gout should be much lower than it was in the clinical trials. If it is important to regulate blood pressure with a diuretic and uric acid levels rise to > 10 mg % or gout occurs, the use of allopurinol in doses of 100 to 300 mg/day has generally been effective in reducing the level of hyperuricemia and preventing gout.

■ Hypercalcemia

Hypercalcemia may also occur in a small number of patients because the use of diuretics results in calcium retention. This has not proved to be a problem, however, but in some instances, has led to additional testing to rule out hyperparathyroidism. An elevation of calcium levels may represent an advantage in some osteoporotic individuals, especially postmenopausal women. There is some evidence, although it is not conclusive, that the use of thiazide diuretics will prevent osteoporosis and fractures.

Combination Diuretics With Other Medications

Diuretics should remain one of the preferred initial monotherapies. When used in combination with a small dose of a β-adrenergic inhibitor, an ACE inhibitor, angiotensin II receptor antagonist or a CCB, response to normotensive levels is approximately 75% to 80%. There are two combination preparations that have been approved as initial once-a-day therapy:

- Capozide (25 mg captopril/15 mg hydrochlorothiazide)
- Ziac (2.5, 5 or 10 mg bisoprolol/6.25 mg hydrochlorothiazide).

Other effective combination thiazide preparations are also available (Table 5.7). Recent data indicate that combination therapies that contain a diuretic are more effective than those that do not.

Indoline Derivatives

Indapamide (Lozol) is an effective, long-acting diuretic with a chemical composition that differs from that of the thiazides. It is well tolerated and acceptable as a substitute for any of the thiazide diuretics. In the low dosages of 1.25 to 2.5 mg/day presently recommended, any metabolic changes (even short-term) are minimal.

Loop Diuretics

Loop diuretics (ie, furosemide, bumetanide, torsemide and ethacrynic acid) are usually reserved for patients:

- Whose creatinine levels are above 2 mg % (ie, cases where thiazide diuretics may not be effective)
- With congestive heart failure.

These are highly effective diuretics, but in commonly used doses given 2 to 3 times daily, they may not lower blood pressure as much as the longer-acting diuretics. The short duration of action of most of the loop diuretics may explain this effect. *Torsemide* is a longer-acting loop diuretic; blood pressure control has been demonstrated 18 to 24 hours after a single dose. This medication may be as effective on a once-a-day basis in lowering pressure as a thiazide. *Ethacrynic acid* (Edecrin) is a short-acting loop diuretic that can be used in patients who develop a skin rash or photosensitivity to a thiazide; this is the only diuretic that

TABLE 5.7 — SOME AVAILABLE THIAZIDE COMBINATION THERAPIES*
(OTHER THAN POTASSIUM-SPARING DIURETICS)

Generic Name	Trade Name	Lowest Dose Available (mg) (Drug/Thiazide)
atenolol + chlorthalidone	Tenoretic	50/25
benazepril + thiazide	Lotensin HCT	5/6.25
bisoprolol + thiazide†	Ziac	2.5/6.25
captopril + thiazide†	Capozide	25/15
clonidine + chlorthalidone	Combipres	0.1/15
enalapril + thiazide	Vaseretic	5/12.5
lisinopril + thiazide	Prinzide, Zestoretic	10/12.5
losartan + thiazide	Hyzaar	50/12.5
metoprolol + thiazide	Lopressor HCT	50/25

methyldopa + thiazide	Aldoril	250/15
reserpine + chlorthalidone	generic	0.125/25
reserpine + hydralazine + thiazide	Ser-Ap-Es	0.1/25/15
reserpine + thiazide	Hydropres	0.125/25
propranolol + thiazide	Inderide LA	80/50

* All available combinations are not listed.
† Approved as initial once-a-day therapy.

does not contain a sulfur component. Ototoxicity has been noted when this agent is used in large doses.

Metolazone (Zaroxolyn) is a longer-acting, potent diuretic that acts near the proximal tubule; it is effective in the presence of renal insufficiency. We often combine its use in small doses of 1 to 2 mg/day with furosemide or one of the other loop diuretics in difficult-to-manage hypertensive patients with renal disease.

6

β–Adrenergic Receptor Inhibitors

β-Adrenergic receptors inhibit the effect of β-adrenergic stimuli on various organs. *Stimulation* of β-receptors results in:
- Renin release
- Vasodilation
- Bronchodilation
- An increase in pulse rate and cardiac output
- Various metabolic effects such as:
  - An increase in insulin secretion
  - Glycogenolysis
  - Gluconeogenesis in both the liver and skeletal muscle.

β-Adrenergic inhibitors block these effects to various degrees, depending on the specific drug used and the type of β-receptor that is inhibited. For example, they tend to induce:
- Vasoconstriction
- Bronchoconstriction
- A decrease in:
  - Pulse rate
  - Cardiac output
  - Myocardial oxygen demand
  - Blood pressure.

There are several types of β-blockers available (Table 6.1). Acebutolol, atenolol, betaxolol, bisoprolol and metoprolol are more active in inhibiting the action of β_1-receptors on cardiac muscle (cardiac selectivity as well as other smooth muscle sites) than β_2-receptors, which affect peripheral vessels and

TABLE 6.1 — SOME COMMONLY USED β-BLOCKERS FOR TREATING HYPERTENSION*

Generic (Trade) Name	Recommended Dosage Range*		Physiologic Effects	Comments
	Dose (mg)	Frequency		
Atenolol† (Tenormin)	25-100	1/day	→ cardiac output; → plasma renin activity; → blood pressure; → pulse rate	Cardioselective agents may also inhibit β_2-receptors in higher doses (eg, all may aggravate asthma)
Betaxolol† (Kerlone)	5-30	1/day		
Bisoprolol† (Zebeta)	5-10	1/day		
Metoprolol† (Lopressor)	50-200	1 or 2/day		
Nadolol (Corgard)	20-240	1/day		
Propranolol (Inderal)	40-240	2 or 3/day		
Propranolol LA (Inderal LA)	80-160	1/day		

β-Blockers with ISA‡			
Acebutolol† (Sectral)	200-800	2/day	Less effect on heart rate, and vascular and bron-chial smooth muscle	Possible advantage in subjects with bradycardia who must receive a β-blocker—they may produce fewer metabolic effects
Pindolol (Visken)	10-40	2/day		

* As in the other tables, not all available medications are listed. Dosages may also differ from the manufacturer's prescribing information recommendations. These dosages are based on our experience and the belief that if small or moderate doses of one drug prove ineffective, small doses of a medication from another class should be added.

† Cardioselective.

‡ ISA = intrinsic sympathomimetic action (slight β_2-receptor stimulation).

bronchial smooth muscle. Of these agents, bisoprolol appears to possess the greatest degree of cardio-selectivity. Cardiac selectivity theoretically limits β_2-blocker effects on pulmonary function and peripheral vessels. Most investigators, however, agree that even these agents should not be used in:

- Patients with asthma where even a slight block-ade of β_2-agonists may increase asthma
- Patients with severe peripheral arterial disease where even partial blockade of β_2-receptors will leave α- or vasoconstrictor-receptors unop-posed, making peripheral arterial disease worse
- Patients with Raynaud's phenomenon
- (Probably) Patients with insulin-dependent dia-betes.

In general, the cardioselective agents will cause less of a decrease in peripheral flow or pulmonary air movement than nonselective agents, but none are com-pletely "cardioselective."

β-Blockers presumably lower blood pressure by:

- Decreasing cardiac output
- Inhibiting the release of renin
- Possibly reducing norepinephrine release from sympathetic neurons
- Decreasing central vasomotor activity.

Some β-adrenergic inhibitors, such as pindolol (Visken) or acebutolol (Sectral), that have some β_2-agonist or stimulating properties (intrinsic sympatho-mimetic activity [ISA]) may lower blood pressure without:

- Reducing cardiac output
- Producing significant bradycardia.

They may also have less of an effect on peripheral re-sistance; cold extremities are reportedly less common as a side effect. In our experience, however, these agents may be less effective as blood pressure lowering drugs, at least in the dosages that we have used (pindolol [Visken] up to 15 to 20 mg/day, acebutolol [Sectral] up to 400 to 600 mg/day). They are indicated, however, in treating patients with angina or hypertension who have a resting bradycardia, where an additional decrease in heart rate might produce deleterious effects. There are no long-term studies with these specific agents to determine their protective effects in patients with coronary heart disease.

There are also differences in β-blockers regarding their lipid solubility. Those agents that are lipid soluble:

- Cross the blood-brain barrier
- Are reported to produce more central nervous system effects
- Have a shorter duration of action since they are inactivated more rapidly by the liver ("first pass" phenomenon).

Propranolol and metoprolol are examples of lipid-soluble antihypertensive β-blockers.

Atenolol (Tenormin) and nadolol (Corgard) are examples of less lipid-soluble agents; that is:

- Smaller amounts reach the central nervous system
- These agents are more slowly metabolized and are excreted through the kidney
- Their duration of action is longer
- There may be fewer central nervous system side effects.

This, however, is not invariable. In our experience, most of the β-blockers reduce blood pressure to an equal degree, so that choice between the various agents depends on:

- Side effects
- Duration of action
- Tolerability.

β-blockers appear to be:

- Especially effective in young, Caucasian patients
- Especially effective in patients with resting tachycardia
- Preferentially indicated in hypertensive patients with angina or a previous myocardial infarction.

β-Adrenergic inhibitors have been used as either second-step therapy in the clinical trials or as alternative first-step drugs to diuretics in the Heart Attack Primary Prevention in Hypertension (HAPPHY), Metoprolol Atherosclerosis Prevention of Hypertension (MAPHY), Medical Research Council (MRC) in Older Patients, and the Swedish Trial in Older Patients with Hypertension (STOP) studies. In only one of the five large trials have β-blockers been found to reduce the incidence of a first myocardial infarction to a greater degree than diuretics. This study was actually an extension of another trial; interpretation of the results has been questioned. In the MRC in Older Patients Trial, a β-blocker proved less effective than a diuretic in preventing coronary mortality. β-Adrenergic inhibitors have been shown, however, to prevent a second myocardial infarction in patients with known ischemic heart disease and to reduce overall mortality, although this finding has not been noted in all studies (Table 6.2). A meta-analysis of the available data suggests a definite reduction of 20% to 33% in infarctions and overall mortality.

Side Effects

In general, β-adrenergic inhibitors are tolerated well, but some patients develop annoying side effects, especially when these agents are used in large doses (Table 6.3).

■ Pulmonary

Noncardioselective β-blockers may produce symptomatic shortness of breath or asthma in patients who are susceptible to a decrease in air flow. These findings are not common, but occur often enough to warrant a statement that these agents should not be used in a patient with asthma or chronic obstructive pulmonary disease (COPD). Cardioselective β-blockers such as bisoprolol or atenolol may decrease air movement to a somewhat lesser degree. A history of asthma, however, should still be considered a contraindication to the use of any β-adrenergic inhibitor.

■ Cardiac

- *Bradycardia*—It is probably not a good idea to use β-adrenergic inhibitors as initial therapy in patients with resting heart rates of 50 to 55.
- *Fatigue*—The decrease in cardiac output and flow to peripheral muscle groups may result in feelings of fatigue. This is probably the most annoying side effect of the β-blockers, especially in people who are accustomed to vigorous exercise.
- *Decrease in the rate of AV conduction*—This may worsen heart block. β-Blockers should not be used in patients with greater than first-degree heart block.
- *Central effects*—The type of fatigue seen in some patients on β-blockers may be related to a decrease in cardiac output; in other cases, it may be secondary to a central effect. Nightmares, insomnia or vivid dreams may be noted. Although some studies have suggested that depression is a common side effect with β-adrenergic inhibitors, this is not true in our experience, at least in the dosages prescribed. There is some evidence that central nervous

TABLE 6.2 — RESULTS OF β-BLOCKER TRIALS ON TOTAL MORTALITY IN PATIENTS WITH ISCHEMIC HEART DISEASE*

Trial	No. Patients (Randomized)		Mortality		
	Control	Intervention	Control (%)	Intervention (%)	p value[†]
β-Blocker Heart Attack Trial	1921	1916	9.8	7.2	0.005
Multicenter International Study	1520	1533	8.4	6.7	0.051
Lopressor Intervention Trial	1200	1195	5.2	5.5	0.90
Norwegian Multicenter Study	939	945	16.2	10.4	0.0003
Julian et al	583	873	8.9	7.3	0.32
European Infarction Study	880	861	5.1	6.6	0.14
Taylor et al	471	632	10.2	9.5	0.78
Baber et al	365	355	7.4	7.9	0.91
Boissel et al	309	298	11.0	5.7	0.013

Hansteen et al	282	278	13.1	9.0	0.16
Pindolol Study Group	266	263	17.7	17.1	0.36
Anderson et al	242	238	26.2	25.2	0.92
Barber et al	147	151	31.3	27.2	0.51
Wilhelmsson et al	116	114	12.1	6.1	0.18
Ahlmark and Saetre	93	69	11.8	7.2	0.48

* Approximate combined results showed a reduction of: (a) sudden death, 33%; (b) nonfatal infarctions, 20%; (c) overall mortality, 22%; (d) nonsudden death, 20%.

† Significance of mortality reduction.

TABLE 6.3 — SIDE EFFECTS OF β-ADRENERGIC INHIBITORS

Symptoms/Signs	Cautions	Comments
Bradycardia*	Should not be used in patients (a) with heart rate below 50, (b) with more than first degree heart block, or (c) with sick sinus syndrome	Usually not a problem in most people
Fatigue	May indicate adverse effect on cardiac output	Some limitation of exercise tolerance (may be a problem)
Insomnia, bizarre dreams or nightmares	May represent first signs of depression (which does occur in a small number of patients on a β-blocker)	May be less common with cardio-selective agents
Cold hands, exacerbation of Raynaud's phenomenon or increase in symptoms of peripheral arterial disease*	Avoid, if possible, in subjects with definite evidence of peripheral vascular disease or Raynaud's phenomenon	Using small dosages or agents with intrinsic sympathomimetic activity (ISA) may reduce this symptom

Sexual dysfunction	May cause impotence/loss of libido—men; loss of libido/delayed organism—women	May occur in about 5% to 10% of patients
Dyspnea, flare-up of asthma	Avoid in patients with chronic obstructive pulmonary disease or a history of asthma	Unusual in patients without pulmonary disease
Metabolic Changes		
↑ triglycerides, ↓ HDL levels*	Monitor lipids; if definite change occurs, consider other drugs, if possible	Clinical significance of questionable importance
Masks symptoms and signs of hypoglycemia	Probably best to avoid use in insulin-dependent diabetes	Tremor and tachycardia inhibited in insulin shock (sweating intact); recovery delayed
* Less with β-blockers with ISA.		

system effects are less common with the less lipid-soluble β-blockers (eg, atenolol compared with propranolol).

In several comparative studies of β-blockers, diuretics and ACE inhibitors, there were no differences observed in quality-of-life measurements among these drugs (except for propranolol, where quality of life was diminished). In another comparative placebo-controlled study (Treatment of Mild Hypertension Study [TOMHS]) of 5 different classes of drugs, β-blockers and diuretics were both found to improve quality-of-life measurements compared with other medications.

Metabolic Changes Secondary to β-Blockers

- A long-term increase in triglyceride levels and a slight decrease in HDL levels have been noted in patients taking β-blockers without ISA. This effect is less for β-blockers with ISA. The clinical significance of these changes has not been determined.
- As noted, these drugs reduce recurrence of myocardial infarction and mortality in patients with ischemic heart disease.
- Prolonged hypoglycemia may occur in insulin-dependent diabetics who experience an insulin reaction. This phenomenon may actually be seen more commonly in the future in view of recent data suggesting that rigid control of blood glucose levels will reduce cardiovascular risk. More careful control may lead to more frequent insulin reactions; these may be aggravated in some patients taking a β-blocker.
- β-Blocker may mask symptoms of insulin-induced hypoglycemia. Tremor and tachycardia

associated with catecholamine release may be blunted or eliminated by β-adrenergic inhibitors. Sweating is not decreased by the use of these agents. These facts must be considered in any patient on a β-blocker who arrives in the emergency room in coma or semi-coma, with a bradycardia and lacking the usual symptoms of an insulin reaction.

Changes in Renal Blood Flow

In some patients taking β-blockers, there is a decrease in renal blood flow reflecting possible renal vessel constriction. This may not be of great clinical significance, and has not been reported with atenolol or nadolol.

Place in Therapy

β-Blockers have been recommended as one of the first-step drugs in the management of hypertension. Most people tolerate them well, and when β-blockers are used as monotherapy, about 40% to 50% of patients will respond. Blacks respond less well to β-blockers than to diuretics or calcium channel blockers (CCBs), and there is some evidence that the elderly may not respond to as great a degree as younger patients.

In combination with small doses of a diuretic, however, these agents are highly effective in all patient groups with relatively few side effects. This may be one reason for the approval of a bisoprolol-hydrochlorothiazide (HCTZ) combination (Ziac) as initial therapy. While a 6.25 mg dose of HCTZ is effective in only a small percentage of subjects as monotherapy, the number of responders increases significantly when it is combined with the β-blocker. Blood pressure is lowered to goal levels in about 75% to 80% of patients with this type of combination therapy. A β-blocker should be used in almost every post-myocardial infarction patient unless there is a contraindication to its use (eg, pulmonary symptoms, marked bradycardia or heart block, or severe peripheral vascular disease).

7

Combined α_1- and β-Blockers

Two combinations of an α-blocker plus a β-blocker are approved in the United States for use in hypertension (Table 7.1):

- Labetalol (Normodyne, Trandate), which combines a nonspecific β_1- and β_2-blocker with some α_1-blocking activity
- Carvedilol (Coreg), a β-blocker with vasodilatory properties secondary to α_1-blocking activity.

These agents possess a greater degree of β-adrenergic inhibiting activity than α_1-blocking activity. Blood pressure is reduced, mainly as a result of a decrease in peripheral resistance. There is less effect on heart rate and cardiac output than with the β-adrenergic inhibitors alone. Heart rate decreases to only a slight degree; in addition, there is less fluid retention and orthostatic hypotension than with α_1-blockers alone. Changes in renin and catecholamine levels are minimal (Table 7.2).

Labetalol and carvedilol are effective antihypertensive agents. Two of the more common side effects of these drugs are postural hypotension and dizziness, which are noted in between 8% and 10% of patients. These side effects occur not only on initial dosing, but may be noted with increasing dose levels. Fatigue, headache and tingling of the scalp have been reported in about 5% of patients. Titration to an effective dose may be time-consuming, especially with labetalol. This drug has a short duration of action and multiple daily dosing may be necessary. For these reasons,

TABLE 7.1 — COMBINED α_1- AND β-BLOCKERS IN THE TREATMENT OF HYPERTENSION

Generic (Trade) Name	Recommended Dosage Range		Physiologic Effects	Comments
	Dose (mg)	Frequency		
Labetalol (Normodyne, Trandate)	200-500 or 600	2/day	Cardiac output ± ↓, → plasma renin activity, ↓ blood pressure, some decrease in pulse rate	Probably more effective in in Blacks than other β-blockers; may cause postural effects; titration should be based on standing blood pressure
Carvedilol (Coreg)	6.25-25	1 or 2/day	Cardiac output and renal blood flow maintained, blood pressure decreased, antioxidant effects	Beneficial effects in heart failure; may decrease myocardial damage post-myocardial infarction

TABLE 7.2 — PHYSIOLOGIC EFFECTS OF α_1- AND β-ADRENERGIC INHIBITORS

- Blood pressure: ↓
- Heart rate: ↓ but less than with a β-blocker
- Cardiac output: ±, and may decrease in upright position
- Stroke volume: no effect or some increase
- Vascular resistance: ± ↓
- Plasma catecholamines: usually no effect
- Aldosterone and angiotensin II levels: may be decreased
- One of these agents, carvedilol, has potent antioxidant and anti-proliferative effects.

labetalol has not been widely accepted in the United States as a suitable initial agent in treatment. The Sixth Joint National Committee on Detection, Evaluation and Treatment of High Blood Pressure (JNC-VI), however, has recommended this class of medication as a possible alternative for initial treatment.

Part of the problem with labetalol may have been the high dosages that were originally advocated. If a dosage of only 100 mg twice a day is used initially, with an increase to a maximum of only 400 to 500 mg/day, side effects are less frequent (when the drug was introduced, dosages of up to 1200 mg/day were commonly prescribed).

One adverse reaction that is noted with β-blockers is hair loss; this may be less frequent with labetalol. As with other agents, if small doses of a drug in this class are ineffective, combining it with a small dose of a diuretic increases response significantly.

Carvedilol, the newer α_1–β-blocker:

- Has a longer duration of action than labetalol
- In our experience is usually effective in a once-a-day dosage; and

- Titration is relatively simple in the management of hypertension (this may be more difficult in patients with heart failure).

Labetalol and carvedilol are effective in Black patients to a greater degree than some of the β-blockers and lower blood pressure to the same degree as a β-blocker and an α_1-blocker given as two separate medications. Intravenous labetalol has been shown to be useful in the treatment of hypertensive crises or accelerated hypertension. This agent or carvedilol can be used as alternative initial monotherapy, but should be prescribed with caution in the elderly. Titration of blood pressure lowering effects should be based on the levels of standing blood pressure.

Carvedilol has been extensively tested in patients with congestive heart failure who remained symptomatic on an ACE inhibitor, a diuretic and digitalis. Results indicate a definite reduction in morbidity and mortality when this drug is given over and above that achieved with previous "triple-drug therapy." Animal and human studies indicate that carvedilol has antioxidant properties considerably greater than vitamin E, in addition to its β- and α_1-blocking properties. Oxidation of LDL, an essential element in the atherogenic process, is reduced. This may account for the beneficial effects of reducing the degree of myocardial muscle damage in experimental myocardial infarction. This effect and effects on cell proliferation also may be responsible for preventing or delaying the atherogenic process in animal models.

Further studies are under way with this agent, and if its antioxidant (or other properties) are confirmed, carvedilol may present some unique advantages in the treatment of hypertensive patients and patients with ischemic heart disease.

8

Peripheral Adrenergic Inhibitors

The drugs in this class are used infrequently. Two of them, guanethidine (Ismelin) and guanadrel (Hylorel), are highly potent medications and inhibit the activity of the sympathetic nervous system by blocking the exit of norepinephrine from storage granules.

Guanethidine was widely used in the 1950s and 1960s. It is effective on a once-a-day basis even in severe hypertension, and when combined with a diuretic, reduces blood pressure in a high percentage of patients. The occurrence of severe postural hypotension, diarrhea and sexual dysfunction in some patients limits its usefulness. We still use guanethidine in small doses of 10 to 20 mg/day in combination with a diuretic in a few patients who are resistant to other therapy. Unlike some other antihypertensive agents, increasing the dose of guanethidine increases the degree of blood pressure reduction.

Guanadrel is similar to guanethidine, but has a shorter duration of action. Because of this, it is somewhat less potent than guanethidine and is reported to have fewer side effects.

Reserpine acts on the central nervous system by decreasing the transport of norepinephrine into storage granules; eventually the amount of norepinephrine available when nerves are stimulated is reduced. This drug has been in use in the United States since the early 1950s, but had been used as a sedative/tranquilizer/blood pressure lowering agent for many years in eastern European countries and India. When reserpine is given in combination with a diuretic, blood pressure is reduced to goal levels of < 140/90 mm Hg in about 75% to 80% of patients.

Unfortunately, when we used reserpine or its derivatives in the 1950s and early 1960s, dosages that were unnecessarily high (eg, 0.5 to 1 mg/day or more) were given. Side effects, including nasal stuffiness, sedation, and most importantly, depression, were not uncommon. But in those early days of antihypertensive drug treatment, many of us thought that the higher the dose, the better the response, with any of the blood pressure lowering agents. This included the β-blockers (propranolol was given in dosages of up to 3 g/day), hydralazine (often given in dosages up to 1200 mg/day), α-methyldopa (up to 2 to 3 g/day), and even diuretics (up to the equivalent of 200 mg/day of chlorthalidone).

Today, we know that most of these drugs are effective in much smaller dosages. In fact, they have a relatively flat dose-response curve. We still use reserpine *in combination with a diuretic* in some patients (see Table 5.7). It has the advantage of being very inexpensive, and most patients tolerate it well. Physicians should be on the alert, however, for the occasional patient who develops symptoms of depression, such as:

- Fatigue
- Insomnia
- Dreams
- General lack of interest in daily activities, job, etc.

Symptoms may persist for many weeks after the drug is stopped.

Combinations of diuretics with reserpine (Ser-Ap-Es, Hydropres, Diupres) or the whole root rauwolfia (Rauzide) are available (see Table 5.7). Table 8.1 lists dosages and side effects of peripheral adrenergic inhibitors. As with other tables in this book, maximum suggested doses are lower than those given in the

TABLE 8.1 — PERIPHERAL-ACTING ADRENERGIC INHIBITORS*

Generic (Trade) Name	Recommended Dosage Range		Adverse Reactions	Physiologic Effects	Comments
	Dose (mg)	Frequency			
Guanadrel* (Hylorel)	10-20	2/day	Sexual dysfunction, dizziness, diarrhea	Inhibits catecholamine release from neuronal storage sites	May cause orthostatic and exercise-induced hypotension
Guanethidine* (Ismelin)	10-20	1/day			
Rauwolfia Alkaloids					
Rauwolfia serpentina*	50-100	1/day	Depression, nasal stuffiness, activation of peptic ulcer	Depletion of tissue stores of catecholamines	Depression may persist for weeks following discontinuation of drug
Reserpine					
Reserpine*	0.05-0.1	1/day			
Reserpine combinations	See Table 5.7	1/day			

* These agents are used infrequently, but may be helpful in some cases, especially when used in combination with a diuretic.

8

manufacturer's prescribing information. This modification is based on long experience and the fact that most of these drugs are used in combination with a diuretic.

9

Central Agonists

The central agonists have an unusual mechanism of action in the vasomotor centers of the brain. By stimulating α_2-receptors, they stimulate inhibitory neurons and decrease sympathetic outflow from the central nervous system. Their hemodynamic effects include:

- A decrease in peripheral resistance
- A slight decrease in cardiac output
- A decrease in blood pressure.

Among the available central agonists are:

- α-methyldopa (Aldomet)
- Clonidine (Catapres)
- Guanabenz (Wytensin)
- Guanfacine (Tenex).

9

These medications reduce blood pressure to normotensive levels in about 35% to 50% of patients, and in combination with small doses of a diuretic, are even more effective.

But side effects occur in a high percentage of patients and dropout rates from therapy can be as high as 20% to 30%. In addition, studies have shown that quality-of-life measurements are decreased more when these drugs are used than when diuretics, ACE inhibitors, most β-blockers or calcium channel blockers (CCBs) are given. Table 9.1 lists these agents, along with their physiologic effects and adverse reactions. The most common side effects include:

- Sedation
- Dry mouth
- Drowsiness

TABLE 9.1 — CENTRAL AGONISTS

Generic (Trade) Name	Recommended Dosage Range		Adverse Reactions	Physiologic Effects	Comments
	Dose (mg)	Frequency			
Clonidine (Catapres)	0.1-0.8	2/day	Dry mouth, drowsiness, headache, fatigue, depression	Stimulate central α_2-receptors that inhibit efferent sympathetic activity—blood pressure ↓; peripheral resistance ↓; no significant effect on heart rate, CO, renal blood flow or G.F.R.	Clonidine patch is replaced once a week. None of these agents should be withdrawn abruptly because of rebound hypertension
Clonidine (Catapres-TTS [patch])	01.-0.2	1/week			
Guanabenz (Wytensin)	4-16	2/day			
Guanfacine (Tenex)	1-3	1/day			
Methyldopa (Aldomet)	250-1000	2/day	Possible immune reactions		

- Dizziness
- Fatigue
- Headaches
- Depression
- Dreams.

Symptoms of depression may be subtle, as they are with reserpine, and include a decrease in mental alertness, vivid dreams, or a decrease in the ability to enjoy life.

In addition to the above adverse effects, which are shared by methyldopa, clonidine, guanabenz and guanfacine, methyldopa may induce certain autoimmune disorders. Abnormal liver function tests and fever may occur in 5% to 10% of patients, and a positive Coombs' test in as many as 35% to 40% of patients. Hemolytic anemia, however, is uncommon.

There are many patients who have done well on methyldopa (usually in combination with a diuretic) for years, with normal blood pressures, few side effects, and no evidence of an autoimmune reaction. In these patients, there is no reason to change therapy. Dosages should probably not exceed 750 to 1000 mg/day. Dosages closer to the starting range (ie, 250 mg/day) should be used in combination with a diuretic when methyldopa is begun.

Clonidine is similar in action to α-methyldopa, with a somewhat shorter duration of action. It can be absorbed through the skin and is available as a transdermal patch. The 0.1-mg patch should be changed every 7 days. Local skin reactions occur in as many as 30% of patients with the transdermal patch. When used orally, the initial dosage of clonidine should be 0.1 mg twice a day increasing to a maximum dosage of 0.3 or 0.4 mg twice a day. Small doses of a diuretic should probably be used with clonidine to increase effectiveness and reduce side effects rather than increase the dosage to higher levels.

9

Drowsiness, dry mouth and fatigue are the most common side effects with clonidine therapy. Use of the patch may result in fewer adverse reactions. A deterrent to the widespread use of clonidine is the fact that if the drug is stopped, the sympathetic nervous system becomes overactive from a suppressed state; there can be a marked overshoot in blood pressure with episodes of severe hypertension. This diagnosis should be considered in any patient who abruptly stops clonidine therapy; restarting the drug will reduce blood pressure. The clonidine patch has also been used in the treatment of nicotine addiction with varying results.

Guanabenz is similar to clonidine. Starting dosages are about 2 to 4 mg twice a day; the maximum dosage should probably not exceed 16 mg/day. Guanfacine (Tenex) is also similar, with a dosage range of 1 to 3 mg/day (Table 9.1).

The use of this class of drugs has decreased in recent years because of the availability of medications that are better tolerated. However, some possible indications for central agonists are:

- Insulin-dependent diabetics
- Patients with asthma or those with peripheral arterial disease where a β-blocker should probably not be used
- In patients who have experienced annoying side effects with ACE inhibitors (angioedema, cough, loss of taste, etc.) or CCBs (palpitations, dizziness, persistent edema, constipation, etc.)
- As a third-step medication in patients who have not responded to other agents.

Methyldopa is still used in treating the hypertension of toxemia of pregnancy. Details of management of this entity can be found in any standard textbook on hypertension.

10 α₁-Adrenergic Inhibitors

At present, there are three α_1-blockers available in the United States:

- Doxazosin (Cardura)
- Prazosin (Minipress)
- Terazosin (Hytrin).

These drugs act by blocking or inhibiting the post-synaptic α_1-receptors on vascular smooth muscle. This inhibits the uptake of catecholamines by smooth muscle cells. Vasoconstriction is blunted, and peripheral vasodilation occurs (Figure 10.1).

There are also several nonselective α-blockers available, ie, phentolamine (Regitine) and phenoxybenzamine (Dibenzyline). These agents block not only the postsynaptic α_1-receptors, but also the presynaptic α_2-receptors located on the neuronal membrane itself. These drugs have not proved effective for the long-term management of hypertension. Although they reduce blood pressure (often dramatically), their action on α_2-receptors removes an inhibiting effect on norepinephrine release; more of this substance is released into the circulation, tachycardia occurs, and tachyphylaxis to blood pressure lowering follows fairly quickly. In addition, postural hypotension and other adverse reactions mitigate against the use of these agents, except in the therapy of pheochromocytoma where they are highly effective.

Although recent studies have shown that the α_1-receptor blockers (prazosin, terazosin and doxazosin) reduce diastolic pressure to as great an extent as other classes of antihypertensive drugs, our experience suggests that their effect on systolic blood pressure is

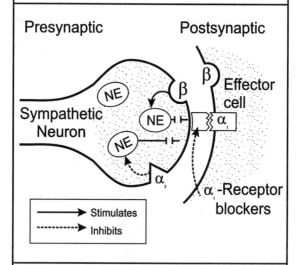

FIGURE 10.1 — MODE OF ACTION OF α_1-BLOCKERS

Presynaptic

Postsynaptic

Sympathetic Neuron

NE

Effector cell

β

α_2

α_1-Receptor blockers

→ Stimulates

-----> Inhibits

Abbreviations: NE, norepinephrine.

A schematic representation of a neuron and a vascular smooth muscle cell showing how α_1-blockers preferentially block the α_1-receptor and leave the presynaptic α_2-receptor unblocked.

Adapted from: Kaplan NM. *Clinical Hypertension*, 5th ed. Baltimore, Md: Williams & Wilkins; 1990:211.

somewhat less. In addition, symptomatic side effects occur in a higher percentage of patients than with some of the other drugs. For example, in a 1-year study of an α_1-receptor blocker (prazosin), 18 of 42 patients dropped out of therapy because of adverse reactions. In a comparative study, only three patients on hydrochlorothiazide discontinued therapy. Side effects of α_1-receptor blockers include:

- Postural hypotension
- Tachycardia

- Dizziness
- Occasional gastrointestinal distress.

Postural hypotension and dizziness may occur on initiation of therapy or on any increase in dosage. These side effects are less common with the longer-acting α_1-blocker doxazosin (Cardura). Dosage should be started at 1 mg/day at bedtime and gradually titrated to a maximum of 5 mg bid. We usually use an α_1-blocker such as doxazosin (Cardura), as a third-step drug in combination with a diuretic and β-adrenergic inhibitor. Dosages are kept to a minimum, which results in fewer and more tolerable side effects. These agents are particularly effective in reducing diastolic blood pressure if this has not been brought to normotensive levels with other medications. Table 10.1 reviews actions, side effects and dosages of α_1-receptor blockers.

Several trials have demonstrated that α_1-receptor blockers may have a favorable effect on lipid levels. In comparative studies with four other medications, doxazosin was shown to decrease cholesterol levels and raise HDL levels to a greater degree than other agents (Table 10.2). In addition, there is some evidence that these drugs will reduce plasma insulin levels and improve glucose tolerance (not all studies have confirmed this). Because of these possible advantages, it has been suggested that the α_1-blockers may be ideal antihypertensive agents. However, because a complicated titration regimen may be required and symptomatic adverse reactions are fairly common, α_1-blockers have not been widely accepted by physicians as Step-I therapy. The addition of an α_1-blocker such as doxazosin to a β-adrenergic inhibitor (which may raise serum triglycerides and, in some instances, reduce HDL levels) is a reasonable approach to therapy. Similar results may be achieved in some patients by using a combined β- and α_1-blocker such as labetalol

TABLE 10.1 — α_1-RECEPTOR BLOCKERS

Generic (Trade) Name	Recommended Dosage Range		Adverse Reactions	Physiologic Effects	Comments
	Dose (mg)	Frequency			
Doxazosin (Cardura)	1.0-10	1/day	Dizziness, palpitations, GI disturbances	Block postsynaptic α_1-receptors—vasodilation—peripheral resistance $\downarrow$; BP $\downarrow$	All may cause postural effects; titration should be based on standing blood pressure
Prazosin (Minipress)	1.0-10	2 or 3/day			
Terazosin (Hytrin)	1.0-10	1-3/day			

Abbreviations: BP, blood pressure.

TABLE 10.2 — AVERAGE CHANGE FROM BASELINE IN PLASMA LIPIDS IN TREATMENT OF MILD HYPERTENSION STUDY (TOMHS) AT 4 YEARS

Lipids (mg/dL)	Acebutolol	Amlodipine	Chlorthalidone	Doxazosin	Enalapril	Placebo
Total cholesterol	-11.7	-6.7	-4.5	-13.8	-8.0	-5.1
LDL cholesterol	-10.6	-5.1	-3.6	-11.3	-5.9	-3.6
HDL cholesterol	0.2	2.0	2.1	2.4	2.6	1.4
Triglycerides	-6.4	-18.4	-14.7	-24.9	-23.6	-14.5

Abbreviations: LDL, low-density lipoprotein; HDL, high-density lipoprotein.

From: Neaton JD, et al. *JAMA*. 1993;270:713-724.

or carvedilol. The α_1-blockers have a favorable effect on symptoms of prostatic hypertrophy and are useful in the management of older hypertensive men with this problem.

11 Direct Vasodilators

Two vasodilators, hydralazine (Apresoline) and minoxidil (Loniten) have been available for the treatment of hypertension for many years. They act directly on vascular smooth muscle (as potassium channel openers?). Hydralazine was used for many years in combination with reserpine and a diuretic; later, in the 1950s and 1960s, it was used as a third-step drug with a β-blocker and a diuretic. These combinations effectively lowered blood pressure in a high percentage of patients, even those with severe hypertension. Diastolic pressure is often reduced more effectively when hydralazine is added to other drugs.

As a result of dilation of arterioles with a decrease in peripheral resistance and blood pressure, baroreceptors are stimulated; an increase in heart rate and release of catecholamines results (Table 11.1). This may lead to renal retention of sodium with expansion of fluid volume. Because of these effects, hydralazine or minoxidil alone may be only temporarily effective as a blood pressure lowering agent. Tachyphylaxis to their effects develops rapidly. Side effects such as the following also limit their usefulness as monotherapeutic agents:

- Tachycardia
- Fluid retention
- Flushing
- Headaches
- In the case of minoxidil, excessive hair growth, not just on the face but on the body. This is especially troublesome in women, and the drug should probably not be used in women except in the rare case of severe hypertension that is

TABLE 11.1 — PROPERTIES OF AVAILABLE DIRECT VASODILATORS

Generic (Trade) Name	Recommended Dosage Range		Adverse Reactions	Physiologic Effects	Comments
	Dose (mg)	Frequency			
Hydralazine (Apresoline)	50-300	2-4/day	Tachycardia, flushing, headaches, fluid retention, lupus-like reaction	Direct smooth muscle vasodilation (primarily arteriolar)	Subject to phenotypically determined metabolism (acetylation)
Minoxidil (Loniten)	2.5-80	1 or 2/day	Tachycardia, flushing, headaches, fluid retention, excessive hair growth	See hydralazine	Both agents: Should use with a diuretic and β-blocker to minimize fluid retention and reflex tachycardia

resistant to multiple drug therapy (eg, renal insufficiency).

The compensatory mechanism that prevents long-term blood pressure lowering and produces side effects may be mitigated by the concurrent use of an adrenergic-inhibitor such as reserpine or clonidine, or a β-blocker. In patients on minoxidil, large doses of a potent diuretic may have to be used to prevent the massive accumulation of fluid that may occur. In these cases, drugs such as furosemide (Lasix) may be needed in dosages of up to 200 mg/day or more, metolazone (Zaroxolyn or Diulo) in dosages of up to 10 mg/day, or torsemide (Demadex) in dosages of up to 15 to 20 mg a day.

We currently prescribe hydralazine infrequently and prefer an α_1-blocker as a third drug. However, in some patients who do not respond to a diuretic plus a β-blocker, hydralazine may be useful in an approximate starting dosage of 25 mg twice a day, increasing to about 100 to 150 mg twice a day. We rarely use dosages higher than these because a lupus-like syndrome may occur on higher doses. This is not common, but positive antinuclear antibody (ANA) tests may occur in as many as 40% of patients. If a patient who is taking hydralazine does develop a fever, rash or arthralgias, the drug should be stopped and other drugs substituted.

Minoxidil is rarely, if ever, used as initial therapy and its use is limited to patients with severe hypertension and renal insufficiency, or patients resistant to or unable to tolerate other medications. As noted, fluid retention and hirsutism are the most commonly noted side effects.

Although direct vasodilators are highly effective antihypertensive drugs, there is little or no place for them as initial monotherapy and other drugs have largely taken their place, ie, ACE inhibitors, angio-

113

tensin II receptor antagonists, calcium channel blockers (CCBs), and α_1-adrenergic inhibitors. Hydralazine is useful in some cases of accelerated or malignant hypertension or in toxemia of pregnancy. Table 11.2 lists possible indications for the use of this drug.

TABLE 11.2 — WHEN TO USE HYDRALAZINE (APRESOLINE)

- In patients with or without renal insufficiency, if blood pressure is not normalized by a diuretic plus a β-blocker or an ACE inhibitor, or a diuretic plus reserpine
- As part of therapy for malignant or accelerated hypertension when there is a reason not to use a CCB, an ACE inhibitor, or an angiotensin II receptor antagonist
- Intravenously in a hypertensive crisis or pre-eclampsia.

---

12   ACE Inhibitors

Angiotensin converting enzyme (ACE) inhibitors are among the most effective vasodilating antihypertensive drugs. These drugs prevent the conversion of angiotensin I, an inactive octapeptide, to angiotensin II, which is a potent vasoconstrictor and aldosterone stimulator (Figure 12.1). In addition, ACE inhibitors prevent the degradation of bradykinin (a vasodilator substance) by inhibiting kininase II, an enzyme that inactivates bradykinin. Bradykinin levels are increased, enhancing the synthesis of various prostaglandins (which also act as vasodilators). Thus, ACE inhibitors have a combined action of decreasing the generation of angiotensin II and increasing the levels of bradykinin and various prostaglandins.

ACE inhibitors are effective as monotherapy. In studies comparing five different classes of drugs, blood pressure reduction with ACE inhibitors was essentially equivalent to that of the other medications, except in Black patients who were less responsive. A list of some of the ACE inhibitors presently available in the United States is given in Table 12.1. Others are under investigation. Most ACE inhibitors have similar actions although they differ chemically. Some contain a sulfhydryl group (like captopril [Capoten]). This may be a factor in causing some of this drug's side effects, such as loss of taste; however, this has not been proven.

ACE inhibitors differ in duration of action and mode of excretion and, therefore, in frequency of administration. They produce some degree of natriuresis and potassium retention as a result of decreasing aldosterone secretion. Blood pressure decreases because of vasodilation and reduction in peripheral re-

FIGURE 12.1—SITE OF ACTION OF ACE INHIBITORS AND ANGIOTENSIN II RECEPTOR ANTAGONISTS

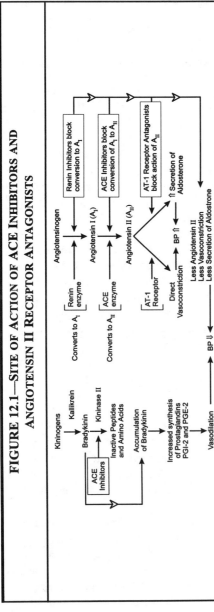

I. Mode of action of ACE inhibitors: block conversion of A_I (an inactive substance) to A_{II} (a vasoconstrictor). This action (1) decreases the generation of A_{II}, and also by blocking the activity of kininase II, (2) decreases the breakdown of bradykinin: this vasodilator substance increases; blood pressure is lowered.

II. Mode of action of angiotensin II (AT-1) receptor antagonists: blocks effects of A_{II}; aldosterone secretion is not increased and vasoconstriction is prevented; *no effect on bradykinin system.*

TABLE 12.1 — ACE INHIBITORS USED FOR TREATING HYPERTENSION

Generic (Trade) Name	Recommended Dosage Range		Adverse Reactions	Physiologic Effects	Comments
	Dose (mg)	Frequency			
Benazepril (Lotensin)	5-20	1 or 2/day	*Cough*, rash, loss of taste, palpitations, rarely angioedema	Blocks formation of angiotensin II, promoting vasodilation and decreased aldosterone; also increases bradykinin and vasodilator prostaglandins	Diuretic doses should be reduced before starting ACE inhibitor whenever possible to prevent excessive hypotension. Reduce dose in patients with serum creatinine > 2.5 mg/dL. May cause hyperkalemia in patients with renal impairment or in those receiving potassium-sparing agents. Can cause renal failure in patients with bilateral renal artery stenosis
Captopril (Capoten)	12.5-150	2/day			
Enalapril (Vasotec)	2.5-20	1 or 2/day			
Fosinopril (Monopril)	5-20	1 or 2/day			
Lisinopril (Zestril, Prinivil)	5-20	1/day			
Moexipril (Univasc)	7.5-15	2 qd			
Quinapril (Accupril)	5-20	1 or 2/day			
Ramipril (Altace)	1.25-10	1 or 2/day			
Trandolapril (Mavik)	1-4	1 qd			

12

sistance. Cardiac output is not decreased and, despite the decrease in blood pressure, there is usually only a slight increase in heart rate. We have, however, seen some patients who develop a persistent low grade tachycardia following the use of an ACE inhibitor.

The ACE inhibitors are particularly effective as unloading agents in the treatment of heart failure because of the reduction in afterload. In addition, in heart failure the levels of angiotensin II are high; reducing these levels is beneficial and may have a favorable effect on cardiac function over and above the effect on vascular resistance. In long-term studies, patients with heart failure have improved in exercise tolerance and other symptoms following the addition of an ACE inhibitor to standard therapy with digitalis and diuretics. In addition, morbidity and mortality have been reduced. Mortality from recurrent myocardial infarction has also been reduced by the use of ACE inhibitors in patients with ischemic heart disease and reduced left ventricular function (ejection fractions below 40%).

ACE inhibitors are one of the groups of drugs suggested as first-step therapy in special situations by the Sixth Joint National Committee (JNC-VI). Long-term studies have not been done to demonstrate a reduction of morbidity and mortality in hypertensive patients when these drugs are used, but several such trials are underway. As noted, it is probable that they will demonstrate that ACE inhibitors are as effective as the drugs that have thus far been tested (ie, diuretics and β-blockers). In one study (SOLVD) in a subset of hypertensive subjects with decreased ejection fractions, the use of ACE inhibitors decreased the incidence of congestive heart failure but not the occurrence of angina or myocardial infarction.

If an ACE inhibitor is used as first-step monotherapy, small doses should be prescribed initially (Table 12.1); the maximum suggested doses in this table may be lower than those recommended in the manufacturer's prescribing information. Rather than increase dosage to a maximum, we prefer to add a small dose of a diuretic if target blood pressure is not achieved with a minimal or, at most, moderate dose of an ACE inhibitor. This approach is similar to our approach to therapy with other medications. For example, if a patient is taking 10 mg/ day of enalapril (Vasotec) or lisinopril (Zestril), or 50 mg/day of captopril (Capoten) and blood pressure has not normalized, a diuretic should probably be added. Here is another instance where combination therapy with one of the many available medications should be considered. Several combinations of an ACE inhibitor and a diuretic are available (see Table 5.7).

Side Effects

Side effects of the ACE inhibitors are relatively uncommon, except for cough. Most patients tolerate ACE inhibitors well and quality of life is not compromised; in fact, some people clearly feel better on these agents. Several adverse reactions have been noted:

- About 15% to 20% of patients develop a dry, hacking cough that is persistent and annoying. If it is recognized early, patients can be saved the trouble of going through extensive diagnostic evaluations for various types of allergies, bronchitis or pulmonary disease. The cough will usually, but not always, disappear in 3 to 5 days on cessation of the medication. It is reported to be more common in women, but in our experience, almost an equal number of men and women develop it. The etiology is unknown, but it may be related to increased levels of bradykinin or substance P. The fact that cough is rare in patients receiving an angiotensin II receptor antagonist that has no effect on the bradykinin system is good evidence that excess bradykinin is related to this adverse effect.

- Postural hypotension and dizziness may occur, especially in patients already receiving a diuretic (this is actually not a common occurrence).
- Angioedema is rare, but can be serious; there is an acute onset of difficulty in breathing or swallowing. This reaction has occurred in three of our patients. It usually occurs within several days to 1 week of institution of therapy and normally clears quickly.
- A macular rash is occasionally seen (about 3% to 5% of cases).
- Loss of taste and appetite is uncommon, but does occur, especially in older people. Symptoms can be subtle and weight loss can result if medicine is not stopped within a short time. It may take more than 2 weeks for taste to return to normal.

Although the manufacturer's prescribing information suggests that diuretics be stopped prior to the addition of an ACE inhibitor, we follow a different strategy. We may reduce the diuretic dosage to about one-half and start the ACE inhibitor in small doses. In some cases, measures of renal function (ie, blood urea nitrogen [BUN] or creatinine levels) rise following the institution of therapy with an ACE inhibitor, especially if a diuretic is being used concurrently. This occurs not only in patients with bilateral renal artery stenosis but also in others, especially older people who undoubtedly have some nephrosclerotic changes.

In patients with bilateral narrowing of the renal arteries and renovascular hypertension, blood pressures often are dependent on high levels of angiotensin

II (a decrease in renal blood flow from the stenosis increases renin release, which leads to an increase in angiotensin II in an attempt to maintain an adequate pressure and flow in the renal arteries). The decrease in blood pressure and intrarenal pressure brought about by ACE therapy may significantly reduce renal blood flow. Simple measures of renal function (ie, BUN and creatinine levels) should be checked within 1 to 2 months after beginning ACE inhibitor therapy; if a *marked* change occurs, therapy should be reevaluated.

Although it was originally believed that ACE inhibitors would only be effective in hypertensive patients with high renin levels, this has not proved to be true. Although these medications are more effective in patients with high-renin hypertension (about 15% to 20% of all hypertensives), they will also lower blood pressure in many patients with normal or low renin levels. As noted elsewhere (see Section 2, *Diagnosis*), measurement of renin levels has not been recommended as an initial diagnostic procedure. We find it of very little value in choosing an appropriate mode of therapy.

ACE inhibitors have been found to be especially effective as antihypertensive agents in young or middle-aged Caucasians. They are less effective in Blacks and in some instances may be less effective in the elderly. The combination of an ACE inhibitor with a small dose of a diuretic is, however, highly effective in young and old, Black and Caucasian patients.

Recent data have demonstrated that ACE inhibitors may decrease insulin resistance. This effect provides a possible theoretic reason to use these agents preferentially in certain subsets of patients (eg, those who are obese, or have elevated triglyceride levels and low HDL levels). These patients probably have increased insulin resistance and are at risk for type II diabetes. The use of an ACE inhibitor (most often with a diuretic and/or a β-blocker) will slow down progression of renal failure in subjects with type I diabetic neuropathy. These agents should be considered drugs of choice in these patients.

Normal blood pressure levels will be achieved in about 30% to 40% of patients with Stage I or Stage II hypertension when an ACE inhibitor is used as monotherapy. However, when a small dose of a diuretic is added to the ACE inhibitor, goal blood pressures of < 140/90 mm Hg will be achieved in approximately 75% to 80% of patients, regardless of race or age.

The ACE inhibitors represent a major advance in the management of hypertension. Their availability has led to an increased rate of control and has simplified management of many patients. We have used the ACE inhibitors most often in combination with a diuretic.

13 Angiotensin II Receptor Antagonists

Numerous agents that block or inhibit the renin-angiotensin-aldosterone system at various sites (Figure 12.1) are being developed. Renin inhibitors, as well as many different angiotensin II inhibitors, are presently under investigation.

Several angiotensin II inhibitors have been approved by the FDA (see Table 13.1): losartan (Cozaar), valsartan (Diovan) and irbesartan (Avapro). Most studies indicate that these medications are as effective in lowering blood pressure as the ACE inhibitors when used as monotherapy. They are well tolerated and have the advantage of lowering blood pressure without the problem of cough. The angiotensin II receptor antagonists block the effect of angiotensin II on blood vessel walls and do not interfere with the breakdown of bradykinin.

The angiotensin II-blocking drugs may interfere with other pathways since angiotensin II is not generated solely by the renin-angiotensin system. The exact significance of this effect is unknown at this time.

Losartan has been the most extensively studied medication in this group. The use of this agent results in an increase in the excretion of uric acid. An increase in serum potassium is infrequent although this effect would have been expected because of the decrease in aldosterone production. Losartan has been shown to reduce mortality, primarily due to sudden death, to a greater degree than an ACE inhibitor in patients with congestive heart failure. In addition, some data suggest that it produces beneficial effects in diabetic nephropathy and in patients with micro-

TABLE 13.1—ANGIOTENSIN II RECEPTOR ANTAGONISTS USED FOR TREATING HYPERTENSION

| Generic (Trade) Name | Recommended Dosage Range | | Adverse Reactions | Physiologic Effects | Comments |
	Dose (mg)	Frequency			
Losartan (Cozaar)	50-100	1/day	Occasional dizziness; generally well tolerated	Blocks action of angiotensin II; → vasodilation; ↓ aldosterone secretion	Diuretic doses should be reduced before starting angiotensin II receptor antagonists whenever possible to prevent excessive hypotension. Reduce dose in patients with serum creatinine > 2.5 mg/dL. Can cause renal failure in patients with bilateral renal artery stenosis
Valsartan (Diovan)	80-320	1/day			
Irbesartan (Avapro)	150-300	1/day			

proteinuria. Studies in specific patient populations with the other medications in this group are ongoing.

The blood pressure lowering effects of the angiotensin II receptor antagonists, as with the ACE inhibitors, are greatly increased when a diuretic is added. A fixed-dose combination of losartan (50 mg) and hydrochlorothiazide (12.5 mg) (Hyzaar) is available and effective in lowering blood pressure in both Black and Caucasian patients, and in the young and elderly. This combination may be appropriate initial therapy in many hypertensive patients.

Long-term morbidity/mortality studies are also underway with these agents in hypertensive patients.

13

14 Calcium Channel Blockers

In the past 15 to 20 years, numerous calcium channel blockers (CCBs) have been introduced; a list of many of these appears in Table 14.1. The CCBs lower blood pressure by inhibiting the entry of calcium ions into vascular smooth muscle cells, which:

- Reduces vascular tone and contractility
- Results in vasodilation
- Reduces peripheral resistance
- Decreases blood pressure.

There are several types of CCBs. The nondihydropyridines diltiazem (Cardizem CD and SR, Dilacor XR, Tiazac), verapamil (Calan SR, Isoptin SR, Verelan, Covera-HS) and mibefradil (Posicor) act on heart muscle as well as peripheral arterioles. Some of these agents, especially the verapamil types of CCBs, may result in partial blockade of the atrioventricular (AV) or sinoatrial (SA) node, as well as have a negative inotropic effect. Sinus rate may be slowed and degree of heart block increased. In addition to lowering blood pressure, the nondihydropyridine CCBs may be useful in the treatment of cardiac arrhythmias, especially in the treatment of supraventricular arrhythmias. Because of negative inotropic effects, however, left ventricular systolic function may be adversely affected and congestive heart failure may result in patients with ischemic heart disease. This is uncommon, but is more likely to occur if this type of CCB is given in combination with a β-blocker. The long-acting formulations of diltiazem (Cardizem CD, Dilacor XR, Tiazac) and verapamil (Calan SR,

TABLE 14.1 — CALCIUM CHANNEL BLOCKERS

Generic (Trade) Name	Recommended Dosage Range		Physiologic Effects	Comments and Probable Side Effects
	Dose (mg)	Frequency		
Diltiazem SR (Cardizem SR)	120-360	2/day	Block inward movement of calcium ions across cell membranes and cause smooth-muscle relaxation. Peripheral resistance ↓; BP ↓; heart rate ↔↓	Block slow channels in heart and may reduce sinus rate; increase degree of arteriovenous block; constipation
Diltiazem CD (Cardizem CD, Dilacor XR, Tiazac)	120-360	1/day		
Verapamil LA (Calan SR, Covera-HS, Isoptin SR, Verelan)	90-360	1-2/day		
Mibefradil (Posicor)	50-100	1/day		

Dihydropyridines				
Amlodipine (Norvasc)	2.5-10	1/day	Block inward movement of calcium ion across cell membranes and cause smooth-muscle relaxation peripheral resistance ↓; BP ↓; heart rate ↔↑	More potent peripheral vasodilators than diltiazem and verapamil, but may cause more dizziness, headache, flushing, peripheral edema, and tachycardia
Felodipine (Plendil SR)	2.5-20	1/day		
Isradipine (DynaCirc CR)	5-20	1/day		
Nicardipine (Cardene SR)	60-90	1/day		
Nifedipine GITS (Procardia XL, Adalat CC)	30-90	1/day		
Nisoldipine (Sular)	20-40	1/day		
Abbreviations: BP, blood pressure.				

14

Isoptin SR, Covera-HS, Verelan) are probably effective when given on a once-a-day basis. Mibefredil (Posicor), a T-channel blocker, is also effective on a once-a-day schedule. At present, the shorter-acting formulations of diltiazem and verapamil are not recommended for therapy.

The dihydropyridine CCBs, such as nifedipine (Procardia, Adalat), nicardipine (Cardene), isradipine (DynaCirc), amlodipine (Norvasc), nisoldipine (Sular) and felodipine (Plendil) act primarily on peripheral vascular beds and have little effect on cardiac muscle contraction or AV conduction. Procardia XL, Adalat CC, Norvasc, Sular, and Plendil SR are probably effective given on a once-a-day basis.

Calcium channel blockers are as effective in reducing blood pressure as the other classes of drugs presently recommended as initial or alternative first-step therapy in the management of hypertension. One study suggests that the percentage of patients achieving a target goal of diastolic blood pressure reduction may be somewhat higher with diltiazem than with other drugs. The CCBs are as effective as diuretics in the elderly and in Black patients and may be more effective than β-adrenergic inhibitors or ACE inhibitors in these individuals.

Calcium channel blockers are effective as monotherapy in Stage I and Stage II hypertension; approximately 35% to 40% of patients will respond. As with other drugs, about 75% to 80% of hypertensive patients will become normotensive when a diuretic and CCB are given together. For example, in one study more than 50% of patients resistant to diltiazem became normotensive when a thiazide was added; more than 50% of patients resistant to a thiazide responded when diltiazem was added. A single combination pill of a CCB and a diuretic is not currently available. Several combination CCBs and ACE inhibitors have recently been approved for use. These combinations are also highly effective; when an ACE inhibitor is given with a dihydropyridine, the degree of edema is decreased. The hypothesis that CCBs will reduce morbidity and mortality in hypertensive patients has not yet been adequately tested.

Adverse Reactions

Side effects differ considerably among the various CCBs. This is not unexpected, given their different sites of action. The dihydropyridine derivatives, felodipine (Plendil), nicardipine (Cardene), nifedipine (Procardia XL), and isradipine (DynaCirc), may cause:

- Flushing
- Headaches
- Postural dizziness
- Palpitations or tachycardia
- Ankle edema.

These reactions are more common with the shorter-acting preparations which should be used with caution or not at all in the treatment of hypertension (see below).

The longer-acting formulations such as nisoldipine and amlodipine may cause fewer side effects than the other agents in this class. Although some studies suggest that reflex tachycardia is not common, an increase in heart rate may occur even with these medications. Ankle edema is especially worrisome to patients who are used to being warned about ankle swelling as a sign of congestive heart failure. Swelling may occur with small doses of any of these compounds and may not respond to diuretics. Edema results from the seepage of fluid from the capillary bed as a result of vasodilation. It usually clears with bed rest. Verapamil may cause severe constipation, postural hypotension, headache and dizziness, and may have a negative inotropic effect on cardiac

14

muscle contraction. Diltiazem may cause headaches and some GI disturbances. Calcium channel blockers have not been shown to have any adverse effects on lipid metabolism or on insulin sensitivity. There is no evidence of any renal functional deterioration when these drugs are used. Some data suggest benefit when these agents are used to treat diabetic neuropathy.

Effects on Coronary Heart Disease

To date, studies with the dihydropyridine CCBs have not shown a significant benefit in preventing a recurrence of myocardial infarction in patients with ischemic heart disease. Some data with short-acting dihydropyridine derivatives suggest that the incidence of myocardial infarctions may actually be increased when these drugs are used. As noted, these agents should be used with caution or not at all in the management of hypertension. A recent 3-year study that compared a diuretic (hydrochlorothiazide) and a dihydropyridine CCB (isradipine) reported a greater incidence of cardiovascular events in the CCB group, primarily new onset angina. It may be that the longer-acting formulations of diltiazem- or verapamil-type CCBs will prove to be more beneficial than the dihydropyridines in reducing CHD. The rate of reinfarction appears to be decreased in patients with ischemic heart disease when verapamil or diltiazem are used.

A recent study suggests that the use of a moderately long-acting dihydropyridine (nitrendipine–not available in the United States) reduced fatal and nonfatal strokes in an elderly population, primarily with isolated systolic hypertension. More data regarding the effects of this class of medication on morbidity and mortality in hypertensive patients will be forthcoming when several ongoing studies are completed.

15   Approach to Therapy

In the 1950s, the treatment of hypertension was fairly simple. The only drugs that had been proved useful and relatively safe were reserpine, hydralazine and diuretics. Others such as the veratrum derivatives and the ganglion-blocking drugs lowered blood pressure, but presented unacceptable side effects in a high percentage of patients. Choices for therapy became more difficult when α-methyldopa, the β-adrenergic inhibitors, peripheral adrenergic inhibitors (eg, guanethidine), and the centrally acting drugs (such as clonidine) became available, but results of therapy were not always satisfactory.

In the past 15 years, treatment has greatly improved with the availability of α_1-receptor blockers, α_1- and β-blockers, ACE inhibitors, calcium channel blockers (CCBs), and angiotensin II receptor antagonists, but choosing the appropriate therapy has often presented a problem. We believe, however, that a simple approach can still be taken in the majority of patients.

There is some rationale for using a type of stepped-care management, although not necessarily the type of stepped-care advocated in 1977 by the First Joint National Committee on Detection, Evaluation and Treatment of High Blood Pressure (JNC-I). Dr. Irvine Page, one of the pioneers in hypertension research, once commented that "stepped-care is merely an attempt to bring order out of chaos." We agree. Stepped-care implies that if blood pressure is not reduced to normal with one drug, it is appropriate to add small doses of another drug from another class. Not all experts concur with this approach and some favor using a sequence of different medications, one at time—if the first is ineffective, stop it and try another, and so on. Our reasons for not favoring this method of therapy are presented below.

The JNC-VI Report issued in 1997 suggests that initial monotherapy should include the use of either a diuretic or a β-adrenergic inhibitor unless there are specific indications for another medication. This recommendation is similar to that of JNC-V in 1993. It is not based on the fact that these drugs are necessarily more effective in reducing blood pressure than other medications, but rather that they are the only drugs that have *thus far* been tested and shown in clinical trials in hypertensive individuals to reduce *cerebrovascular* and *cardiovascular morbidity* and *mortality*.

It is quite possible that other agents (such as the ACE inhibitors, angiotensin II receptor antagonists, and CCBs) that are now being studied in long-term hypertension treatment trials will also be proven to reduce morbidity and mortality. However, at present, there are no data to confirm this. These medications should be considered as alternative therapy or for specific indications. (See Section 4, *Drug Treatment of Hypertension*: *General Information, Specific Drug Therapy* section; and, Tables 4.2, 15.1, 15.2 and 15.3.)

Characteristics of an Ideal Medication for Initial Therapy

Almost all of the available medications satisfy many or most of the criteria of an ideal antihypertensive agent (Table 15.4):

- Most are effective as monotherapy in about 40% to 50% of patients.
- Most can be given on a once-a-day basis with few visits for titration (this may be difficult with some of the shorter-acting α_1-blockers; with the longer-acting α_1-blockers, this is possible).

- Other than the centrally-acting drugs and perhaps some of the α_1-blockers, side effects are not a major problem in the majority of patients. Side effects can be minimized by starting with small doses.
- Although the use of diuretics and β-blockers may result in some changes in lipid levels, these are short-term in the case of diuretics and are of doubtful clinical significance with the β-blockers. The significance of these changes has been overemphasized. It also does not appear at present that the effects of diuretics on insulin resistance are clinically important.
- Long-term effectiveness in lowering blood pressure has been proven with most available anti-hypertensive drugs, but as noted, only two classes of drugs have been shown to reduce both cerebrovascular and cardiovascular morbidity and mortality.
- In the initial choice of drug, cost should be considered. It has been reported that as many as 20% to 25% of patients are unable to afford to fill their prescriptions. It is foolhardy to recommend a drug if the patient is unable to afford it. The two classes of drugs recommended as Step-I agents happen to be the least expensive, but many of the other drugs, such as ACE inhibitors or CCBs, are now available at lower cost than several years ago. If ongoing studies demonstrate that a more expensive medication is more effective than a less costly one, then cost should be considered a secondary issue.

15

TABLE 15.1 — SPECIFIC INDICATIONS AND CONTRAINDICATIONS FOR PARTICULAR ANTIHYPERTENSIVE DRUGS*

Clinical Situation	May Have Favorable Effects	Requires Careful Follow-up	Contraindicated
Cardiovascular			
Angina pectoris	β-Blockers, calcium channel blockers	—	Direct vasodilators
Bradycardia/heart block, sick sinus syndrome	—	—	β-Blockers, labetalol, verapamil, diltiazem
Cardiac failure—systolic dysfunction	Diuretics, ACE inhibitors, A_{II} receptor antagonists, α_1–β-blockers (carvedilol)	—	β-Blockers, calcium channel blockers
Hypertrophic cardiomyopathy with diastolic dysfunction	β-Blockers, diltiazem, verapamil, α_1–β-blockers (carvedilol)	Diuretics	ACE inhibitors, α_1-blockers, hydralazine, minoxidil, A_{II} receptor antagonists
Hyperdynamic circulation (rapid heart rate)	β-Blockers	—	Direct vasodilators
Peripheral vascular occlusive disease	—	β-Blockers	—

	Non-ISA β-blockers, ACE inhibitors (selected patients), verapamil, or diltiazem		Direct vasodilators
After myocardial infarction	Non-ISA β-blockers, ACE inhibitors (selected patients), verapamil, or diltiazem	—	
Renal			
Bilateral renal arterial disease or severe stenosis of artery to solitary kidney	—	—	ACE inhibitors, A_{II} receptor antagonists
Renal insufficiency; early (serum creatinine 1.5-2.5 mg/dL)	—	—	Potassium-sparing agents, potassium supplements
Advanced (serum creatinine ≥ 2.5 mg/dL)	Loop diuretics	ACE inhibitors, diuretics, A_{II} receptor antagonists	Potassium-sparing agents, potassium supplements
Depression	—	$α_2$-Agonists	Reserpine
Diabetes mellitus–Type I (insulin-dependent)	ACE inhibitor/A_{II} receptor antagonists with a diuretic	β-Blockers	—
Diabetes mellitus (with proteinemia)	ACE inhibitor (usually with a diuretic)	Use with caution in patients with serum creatinine > 2.5 mg/dL	—
Liver disease	—	Labetalol	Methyldopa
Vascular headache (migraine)	β-Blockers, non-dihydropyridine CCBs	—	—

* Not all indications or contraindications are listed. See also Tables 15.2 and 15.3.

15

TABLE 15.2 — SPECIFIC INDICATIONS AND CONTRAINDICATIONS FOR PARTICULAR ANTIHYPERTENSIVE DRUGS IN PREGNANCY*

Clinical Situation	Indicated	Requires Careful Follow-up	Contraindicated
Pregnancy			
Preeclampsia	Methyldopa, hydralazine	—	ACE inhibitors, probably A_{II} receptor antagonists
Chronic hypertension	Same medications as prior to pregnancy except ACE inhibitors or A_{II} receptor antagonists	—	ACE inhibitors, probably A_{II} receptor antagonists

* Not all indications or contraindications are listed. See also Tables 15.1 and 15.3.

TABLE 15.3 — INDICATIONS AND CONTRAINDICATIONS FOR INITIAL MONOTHERAPY WITH ANTIHYPERTENSIVE MEDICATIONS*

ACE Inhibitors and Angiotensin II Receptor Antagonists
- Not as effective in Blacks.
- Avoid in patients with bilateral renal artery stenosis and pregnant women.
- Especially useful in congestive heart failure when added to a diuretic and/or digitalis.
- Although some investigators have suggested that ACE inhibitors are not as effective as diuretics in the elderly, there is evidence that both classes of drugs will lower blood pressure in this group of patients.
- May have special use in diabetics or diabetic nephropathy (usually with a diuretic to bring BP levels down to normal).

α_1-Blockers
- May be especially useful in men with prostatic hypertrophy.

β-Blockers
- Less effective in Blacks (may be more effective than diuretics in Caucasians); α_1–β-blockers are effective in both Black and Caucasian populations.
- Avoid in patients with a history of asthma or chronic obstructive pulmonary disease, peripheral arterial disease or marked bradycardia, and possibly in insulin-dependent diabetics. (Compounds with intrinsic sympathomimetic activity may not cause bradycardia.)
- Especially useful in patients with angina.
- The α_1–β-blocker, carvedilol, may be especially useful in resistant congestive heart failure.
- Especially useful in patients with migraine.

Calcium Channel Blockers
- Effective in both Black and Caucasian patients, both young and elderly patients.
- Especially useful in patients with angina.

Diuretics
- Effective in both Black and Caucasian patients, both young and elderly patients.
- Probably should not be used in patients with a history of gout.
- Thiazide diuretics are less effective as antihypertensive agents in the presence of renal insufficiency (> 2.5 mg/dL creatinine). In these instances, a loop diuretic (ie, furosemide, bumetanide, torsemide, ethacrynic acid) or metolazone should be used, probably in combination with other medications.
- May have favorable effect on osteoporosis.

---

* Not all indications and contraindications are listed. See also Tables 15.1 and 15.2.

15

Factors Influencing the Choice of Initial Therapy

The type of treatment program that we prefer to follow uses certain demographic factors in selecting the initial drug:

- White and younger patients (under 50 years of age) generally respond better to an adrenergic inhibitor such as a β-blocker, an ACE inhibitor, or an angiotensin II receptor antagonist. These patients also respond to a diuretic or a CCB, but the percentage of normotensive responders is somewhat lower.
- Older and Black patients respond better to a diuretic or a CCB. Normotensive levels may also be achieved with a β-blocker or an ACE inhibitor, but a smaller percentage of patients become normotensive. The reason for these differences have not been determined. It may or may not be related to pretreatment renin levels. Attempts to define potential responders by measuring plasma renin levels have not been successful.

These general guidelines can be helpful in selecting the Step-I drug. Other factors that are important include:

- If the patient has concomitant diseases such as asthma, insulin-dependent diabetes or definite peripheral arterial disease, a β-blocker usually should not be chosen.

- If a patient has a history of gout, it might be prudent to avoid a diuretic. If blood pressure is not normalized with another medication, a diuretic can be added, but allopurinol may also be necessary to control uric acid levels.

- In patients who are very physically active, β-adrenergic inhibitors may not be a good first choice unless there are specific reasons for their use (eg, angina, migraine headaches).

- In patients with angina, a β-adrenergic inhibitor or a long-acting CCB may be preferred as initial therapy.

- In patients with congestive heart failure or diabetic nephropathy, an ACE inhibitor or an angiotensin II receptor antagonist (plus a diuretic) would be preferred. An $\alpha_1-\beta$-blocker (Carvedilol) may be considered in patients with congestive heart failure (in addition to usual therapy)

- In patients with a previous myocardial infarction, a β-blocker without ISA is preferred.

- Based on evidence (see Section 5, *Diuretics* and Section 6, β-*Adrenergic Receptor Inhibitors*), there is no reason to avoid the use of diuretics or β-blockers in patients with hyperlipidemia and/or hyperglycemia. Although β-blockers may increase triglycerides or reduce HDL over the long term, these effects may not be of clinical importance. Chemical changes should be monitored and the drug stopped or dosage decreased if significant changes occur.

15

Tables 15.1, 15.2 and 15.3 summarize some specific indications and cautions regarding the use of antihypertensive drugs. Table 15.5 outlines characteristics of different antihypertensive medications.

The plan for initial medical therapy that we most often follow is shown in Figure 15.1. This is generally similar to the JNC-VI recommendations, with a few exceptions. A diuretic in small doses equivalent to 12.5 mg of chlorthalidone or 25 mg of hydrochlorothiazide (HCTZ) is given in most patients unless there is a specific contraindication to its use or a specific indication for the use of another agent (see above). A β-blocker is also an acceptable choice for initial therapy. If some blood pressure lowering is noted but normotensive levels are not achieved, dosage will be increased (ie, to 25 mg chlorthalidone or 37.5 to 50 mg of HCTZ). We may use a potassium-sparing thiazide combination (like Dyazide or Maxzide), especially in elderly patients, diabetics or patients receiving digitalis.

If little or no effect is noted from the diuretic, a second drug such as a β-adrenergic inhibitor, an α_1-β-blocker, an ACE inhibitor, an angiotensin II receptor antagonist or, in some cases, a CCB will be added. If a β-blocker was used as initial therapy, a diuretic should be added unless there is a contraindication to its use. In the situation where a patient has been started on an ACE inhibitor or a CCB, a diuretic should be added if normalization of blood pressure has not occurred (dosage ranges for various drugs are listed under the discussion of specific medications).

Multiple Drug Therapy or Sequential Monotherapy?

Using small doses of two different classes of drugs makes good sense, rather than increasing the dosage of one drug to a maximum level. Blood pressure re-

TABLE 15.5 — PHYSIOLOGIC CHARACTERISTICS OF DIFFERENT ANTIHYPERTENSIVE MEDICATIONS*

	ACE/A$_{II}$†	Diuretics‡	β-Blockers	CCBs§	α-Blockers	Centrally Acting Agents	Vasodilators
Peripheral vascular resistance	↓	↓	↑ ↔	↓	↓	↓	↓
Cardiac output	↔	↔	↓	↔	↔	↔	↑
Heart rate	↔ ↑	↔	↓	Variable	↑	↔	↑
Total cholesterol	↔	Short term ↑	↔	↔	↓	↔	↔
LDL cholesterol	↔	Short term ↑	↔	↔	↓	↔	↔
HDL cholesterol	↔	↔	↔ ↓	↔	↔ ↑	↔ ↓	↔
Triglycerides	↔ ↓	↑	↑	↔	↔ ↓	↔ ↑	↔
Race (Black/Caucasian)	Less effective in Blacks	Effective in both	Less effective in Blacks	Effective in both	Effective in both	Probably effective in both	Effective in both

* Most of the available medications reduce peripheral resistance.
† ACE inhibitors and A$_{II}$ receptor antagonists.
‡ Adverse effects on lipid levels are short-term with diuretics—effects on triglycerides and HDL levels with β-blockers are of questionable clinical significance.
§ Calcium channel blockers.

15

143

FIGURE 15.1 — TREATMENT OF HYPERTENSION*

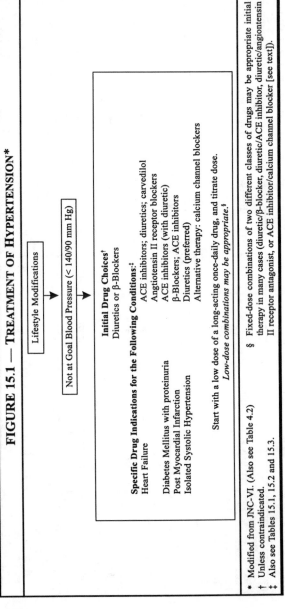

Lifestyle Modifications

↓

Not at Goal Blood Pressure (< 140/90 mm Hg)

↓

Initial Drug Choices[†]
Diuretics or β-Blockers

Specific Drug Indications for the Following Conditions:[‡]

Heart Failure	ACE inhibitors; diuretics; carvedilol
	Angiotensin II receptor blockers
Diabetes Mellitus with proteinuria	ACE inhibitors (with diuretic)
Post Myocardial Infarction	β-Blockers; ACE inhibitors
Isolated Systolic Hypertension	Diuretics (preferred)
	Alternative therapy: calcium channel blockers

Start with a low dose of a long-acting once-daily drug, and titrate dose.
Low-dose combinations may be appropriate.[§]

§ Fixed-dose combinations of two different classes of drugs may be appropriate initial therapy in many cases (diuretic/β-blocker, diuretic/ACE inhibitor, diuretic/angiontensin II receptor antagonist, or ACE inhibitor/calcium channel blocker [see text]).

* Modified from JNC-VI. (Also see Table 4.2)
† Unless contraindicated.
‡ Also see Tables 15.1, 15.2 and 15.3.

sponse is generally better; as noted, about 75% to 80% of patients will respond to a combination of two different agents, whereas only about 50% to 60% will respond even to full doses of one drug. In addition, certain homeostatic reflex mechanisms may be blocked and side effects minimized by this approach. For example, the use of a diuretic will result in increased activity of the renin-angiotensin system, which may possibly prevent the achievement of normotensive levels in some patients. The addition of an ACE inhibitor, angiotensin II receptor antagonist, or a β-blocker will blunt this effect. Studies have shown that both subjective and metabolic adverse reactions are less frequent with smaller doses of medications. The JNC-VI recognizes these benefits of low-dose combination therapy and, as noted, suggests that this approach may be appropriate initial therapy.

With this approach, dosage adjustments and blood pressure monitoring can be at 2 to 3 month intervals in Stage I and, in some cases, Stage II hypertension. In more severe cases, office visits must obviously be more frequent. This also applies if medications produce adverse effects. Once blood pressure is controlled at normotensive levels, patients can be seen only 2 to 3 times a year.

On the other hand, *sequential monotherapy* involves the use of individual drugs, one at time. If one does not work, stop it and try another. This method is expensive, requires more frequent office visits, and is time-consuming, but is advocated by some experts. One disadvantage is that when this type of program is followed, patients may get the feeling that the physician is not quite sure of what s/he is doing, ie, trying one drug, another drug 2 months later, and a third drug 2 months after that. Confidence in therapy is more easily gained if blood pressure reduction is brought about fairly quickly, even if more than one medication has to be used.

15

If blood pressures have been normalized for about 1 year after initiating therapy, it is reasonable to consider withdrawing or reducing the dosage of the first drug (which might not have been effective) to see if the second drug can maintain normotensive levels. It could be argued that if the first drug was relatively ineffective, why not stop it? However, effects on blood pressure of different agents are often additive.

Combination Therapy

Available combinations include diuretics and β-blockers, diuretics and ACE inhibitors, diuretics and angiotensin II receptor antagonists, and ACE inhibitors and CCBs. Using a combination improves efficacy in certain patient groups who may not usually respond to certain agents. For example, in Black patients, an ACE inhibitor or angiotensin II receptor antagonist may be ineffective, and a diuretic may not always lower blood pressure to goal levels; a combination of small doses of one of these drugs with a diuretic is usually highly effective. Some, but not all, of the available antihypertensive medication combinations are listed in Table 15.6.

Figure 15.1 outlines the approach that we follow in most cases of Stage I and, in some cases, Stage II hypertension. In patients with Stage II hypertension, blood pressures of about 160-170/105 mm Hg, especially those with evidence of left ventricular hypertrophy, we may start combination therapy without attempting a period of monotherapy, ie, using a combination of a β-blocker and a diuretic, an ACE inhibitor and a diuretic or an angiotensin II receptor antagonist and a diuretic. This type of treatment may appear to contradict the rule that we have all been taught: not to initiate therapy with several medications. One could argue that if the patient responds, you will not know which drug was effective. This may be true,

146

but does it make a difference if blood pressure is normalized and medication is well tolerated?

To reemphasize, when small doses of two drugs are used instead of large doses of one drug:

- The response rate to therapy is increased from about 40% to 50% to as high as 70% to 80%
- Frequency of office visits may be reduced
- Blood pressure is lowered more quickly
- Side effects are not increased (or are actually minimized)
- Cost is not increased to a great extent.

If blood pressures remain normal after 1 year, one of the agents could be withdrawn. We find this approach to therapy practical in the "real world." JNC-VI has suggested that fixed combination medications are appropriate as initial therapy.

Combination Medications as Initial Therapy

Two fixed combinations of cardioselective β-blockers and diuretics have been approved as initial therapy for hypertension: bisoprolol/hydrochlorothiazide and betaxolol/chlorthalidone. The betaxolol combination is not available at the present time, while the other, bisoprolol/HCTZ (Ziac), is on the market. This medication contains a small dose of the diuretic (6.25 mg) and is available with different dosages of the β-blocker (2.5, 5 and 10 mg). Approval of the drug followed the demonstration that, although the low-dose individual components of the combination were only effective in about 20% to 30% of subjects, the combination lowered blood pressure to goal levels in more than two-thirds of patients. Importantly, because of the small doses of each component, side effects were similar to those of placebo. Placebo-controlled studies have demonstrated that this combina-

15

TABLE 15.6 — SOME AVAILABLE COMBINATION ANTIHYPERTENSIVE MEDICATIONS*

Drug	Trade Name
ACE Inhibitors and Diuretics	
Benazepril 5, 10 or 20 mg/hydrochlorothiazide 6.25, 12.5 or 25 mg	Lotensin HCT
Captopril 25 or 50 mg/hydrochlorothiazide 15 or 25 mg	Capozide†
Enalapril 5 or 10 mg/hydrochlorothiazide 12.5 or 25 mg	Vaseretic
Lisinopril 10 or 20 mg/hydrochlorothiazide 12.5 or 25 mg	Prinzide; Zestoretic
Angiotensin II Receptor Antagonists and Diuretics	
Losartan 50 mg/hydrochlorothiazide 12.5 mg	Hyzaar
β-Adrenergic Blockers and Diuretics	
Atenolol 50 or 100 mg/chlorthalidone 25 mg	Tenoretic
Bisoprolol 2.5, 5 or 10 mg/hydrochlorothiazide 6.25 mg	Ziac†
Metoprolol 50 or 100 mg/hydrochlorothiazide 25 or 50 mg	Lopressor HCT
Nadolol 40 or 80 mg/bendroflumethiazide 5 mg	Corzide
Propranolol (extended release) 80, 120 or 160 mg/hydrochlorothiazide 50 mg	Inderide LA

Calcium Channel Blockers and ACE Inhibitors	
Amlodipine 2.5 or 5 mg/benazepril 10 or 20 mg	Lotrel
Diltiazem 180 mg/enalapril 5 mg	Teczem
Felodipine 5 mg/enalapril 5 mg	Lexxel
Verapamil (extended release) 180 or 240 mg/trandolapril 1, 2 or 4 mg	Tarka
Other Combinations	
Amiloride 5 mg/hydrochlorothiazide 50 mg	Moduretic
Clonidine 0.1, 0.2 or 0.3 mg/chlorthalidone 15 mg	Combipres
Methyldopa 250 or 500 mg/hydrochlorothiazide 15, 25, 30 or 50 mg	Aldoril
Reserpine 0.125 or 0.25 mg/chlorthalidone 25 or 50 mg	Demi-Regroton
Reserpine 0.125 mg/hydrochlorothiazide 25 or 50 mg	Hydropres
Reserpine 0.1 mg/hydralazine 25 mg/hydrochlorothiazide 15 mg	Ser-ap-es
Spironolactone 25 or 50 mg/hydrochlorothiazide 25 or 50 mg	Aldactazide
Triamterene 37.5, 50 or 75 mg/hydrochlorothiazide 25 or 50 mg	Dyazide, Maxzide
* Not all combinations are listed.	
† Approved for initial therapy.	

15

tion is as effective or more effective in lowering blood pressure than an ACE inhibitor (enalapril) or a CCB (amlodipine). In addition, side effects were less frequent with the β-blocker/diuretic combination than with the other medications. An ACE inhibitor/thiazide diuretic combination (capozide) has also been approved for initial therapy. Duration of action of the ACE inhibitor is prolonged when administered with a diuretic.

Some investigators advocate an approach that does not include a diuretic: eg, an ACE inhibitor, if ineffective, add a CCB, or start with a β-blocker and if this is ineffective, add a dihydropyridine CCB. These combinations may be effective, but in our experience, a higher percentage of patients will respond if the treatment regimen includes a diuretic.

16 Results of Therapy

Remarkable progress has been made in the management of hypertension since the 1950s. Figures 16.1 and 16.2 outline the percent decline in age-adjusted mortality since 1972 when the National High Blood Pressure Program was initiated. It should be noted that while noncardiovascular diseases have decreased by only about 12%, death from stroke has decreased by about 55% to 60% in both sexes and in both Black and Caucasian individuals. Not all of this decrease, of course, can be attributed to better control of hypertension since people are smoking less, are more weight conscious, exercise more, and so on. But since hypertension is present in almost 75% of patients with strokes, a good part of the decline can probably be attributed to better management of hypertension. In addition, more than a 50% decrease in coronary heart disease deaths has also been noted; again, in both sexes and in Blacks and Caucasians.

Obviously, as discussed above, there are factors other than better management of hypertension that may account for this dramatic response:
- People are:
  - Smoking less
  - Exercising more
  - Less obese
- The advent of bypass surgery
- Better management of acute coronary events.

16

The results of hypertension treatment are dramatic. There have been 17 major trials since the 1970s. When these are analyzed in Figure 4.1, we see that there has been a:

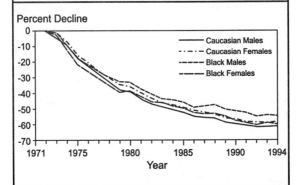

FIGURE 16.1 — PERCENT DECLINE IN AGE-ADJUSTED MORTALITY RATES FOR STROKE BY SEX AND RACE: UNITED STATES, 1972-1994

Percent Decline

— Caucasian Males
-·-·- Caucasian Females
--- Black Males
—— Black Females

Source: *Vital Statistics of the United States*, National Center for Health Statistics.

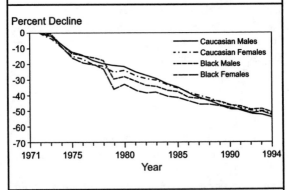

FIGURE 16.2 — PERCENT DECLINE IN AGE-ADJUSTED MORTALITY RATES FOR CHD BY SEX AND RACE: UNITED STATES, 1972-1994

Percent Decline

— Caucasian Males
-·-·- Caucasian Females
--- Black Males
—— Black Females

Abbreviations: CHD, coronary heart disease.

Source: *Vital Statistics of the United States*, National Center for Health Statistics.

- 40% highly statistically significant decrease in stroke morbidity and mortality
- 16% highly statistically significant reduction in coronary heart disease events
- 21% statistically significant decrease in vascular mortality in treated compared to control or placebo subjects.

These trials used diuretics and β-blockers primarily with several other drugs, such as centrally acting or vasodilatory drugs (hydralazine, α-methyldopa and reserpine) being added if no response was noted. None of the trials used ACE inhibitors or calcium channel blockers (CCBs) because they were not available when the studies were launched. However, it is clear that effective lowering of blood pressure with drugs available 15 to 30 years ago has produced excellent results.

In addition, however, to the hard end points of strokes and stroke deaths, myocardial infarctions and myocardial infarction deaths, there are other benefits that have accrued from the effective management of hypertension. Table 16.1 summarizes all of the trials where data were available. These were placebo or controlled trials. It should be noted that 1493 of 13,342 patients in the placebo or control group progressed to more severe disease with systolic pressures higher than 200 to 210 mm Hg and diastolic blood pressures higher than 110 to 120 mm Hg compared with only 95 of 13,389 patients in the treated group. This benefit of therapy represents a "soft end point," but it indicates that early treatment of hypertension prevents progression.

The reversal or prevention of left ventricular hypertrophy has also been noted in clinical trials where data were reported. Table 16.2 shows a highly significant decrease of 35% in the number of patients who developed left ventricular hypertrophy in the treated

16

TABLE 16.1 — EFFECT OF TREATMENT ON PREVENTING PROGRESSION FROM MILD-MODERATE TO MORE SEVERE HYPERTENSION:* FINDINGS FROM MAJOR CLINICAL TRIALS

Study (Range for Mild-Moderate Hypertension—mm Hg)	Placebo		Active Treatment	
	No.	Progressed to More Severe	No.	Progressed to More Severe
USPHS (90-114)	196	24 †	193	0
VA Cooperative (90-114)	194	20	186	0
Australian (95-109)	1706	198	1721	5
Oslo (90-110)‡	379	65	406	1
MRC (90-109)	8654	1011	8700	76
MRC-Elderly (160-209/< 115)	2213	175	2183	13
Total	13,342	1493	13,389	95

Abbreviations: USPHS, US Public Health Service Study; VA, Veterans Administration; MRC, Medical Research Council Study.

* Diastolic blood pressure > 110 mm Hg, systolic blood pressure > 200-210 mm Hg.
† Diastolic blood pressure > 130 mm Hg.
‡ 12.5% of patients had systolic hypertension only.

From: Moser M, Hebert P. *J Am Coll Cardiol.* 1996;27:1214.

TABLE 16.2 — LEFT VENTRICULAR HYPERTROPHY, REPORTED IN RANDOMIZED TRIALS OF BLOOD PRESSURE LOWERING*

	Active Treatment		Control Treatment	
	LVH	No. Randomized	LVH[†]	No. Randomized
Oslo	0	406	7	379
US Public Health Service Study (USPHS)	13	193	25	196
European Working Party on High Blood Pressure in the Elderly (EWPHE)	0	416	1	424
Hypertension Detection and Follow-up Program (HDFP)	127	5135	183	5099
Total: All Trials	140[†]	6150	215	6078

* Not recorded in 11 other trials reviewed.
† Significant reduction of 35% in the occurrence of left ventricular hypertrophy (LVH) in treated compared to control subjects.

From Moser M, Hebert P. *J Am Coll Cardiol.* 1996;27:1214.

16

155

compared to the control group, a classic example of primary prevention. In addition, congestive heart failure (CHF) was dramatically reduced in patients who were actively treated (Table 16.3). A statistically significant decrease of more than 50% in the occurrence of CHF was noted in the clinical trials when treated subjects were compared to controls. These are impressive data, suggesting the importance of the management of hypertension as a measure for the prevention of cardiovascular disease. CHF remains as an increasingly common reason for hospitalization, especially in individuals over 60 years of age. Hypertension, as noted, has been identified as a major factor in the cause of CHF. It is probable that if more hypertensive patients were treated more effectively, the occurrence of CHF would decrease.

Results of Therapy in the Elderly

Finally, more recent studies and several trials in the 1970s and 1980s have shown that these excellent results can be achieved not only in the young, but in the elderly, including patients above 75 or 80 years of age (Table 16.4). Three recent trials have underscored the benefits of treatment of both systolic and diastolic hypertension, as well as isolated systolic hypertension (ISH) in the elderly and have demonstrated not only a decrease in heart failure and stroke, but a decrease in coronary heart disease events as well. One of the trials, the Systolic Hypertension in the Elderly Program (SHEP) (Figure 16.3), employed small doses of a diuretic with a β-blocker added, if necessary, and demonstrated:
- A marked 37% reduction in strokes
- 25% reduction in transient ischemic attacks
- 30% reduction in myocardial infarctions
- 54% reduction in the occurrence of CHF when compared with placebo.

Benefit was noted in diabetic subjects and in patients with hyperlipidemia.

As noted in a recent study (Syst Eur), nitrendipine, a moderately long-acting dihydropyrimidine CCB (not yet available in the United States), was given as initial therapy with an ACE inhibitor or diuretic added, if necessary. Fatal and nonfatal strokes were reduced in elderly patients, primarily with ISH. Confirmatory data are awaited from studies with other CCBs. JNC-VI recommends the use of diuretics as preferred initial therapy in the elderly with ISH. Based on the Syst Eur data, a long-acting dihydropyrimidine may be considered if a diuretic is contraindicated. In our experience, older patients respond well to combinations of small doses of a diuretic/β-blocker, ACE inhibitor or angiontensin II receptor antagonist, diuretic combinations, or a CCB with a diuretic. There are, however, no long-term morbidity-mortality data available at this time for these therapies.

Final Comments

Thus, it would appear that the early, effective and long-term management of hypertension with the agents presently available will reduce not only so-called "hard end points" such as strokes and stroke deaths, myocardial infarctions and CHD death, but also many of the other complications that were previously noted in untreated subjects. The benefit of treatment in prevention of renal insufficiency has not been as carefully tabulated, and there is some concern that patients who are not treated early enough will progress to renal insufficiency.

Further progress must be made in increasing the number of patients with hypertension who are controlled. A recent survey found that only about 50% of patients with hypertension were being treated and that of those who were on therapy, only about one half were controlled at levels below 140/90 mm Hg. Some

16

TABLE 16.3 — CONGESTIVE HEART FAILURE REPORTED IN RANDOMIZED TRIALS OF BLOOD PRESSURE LOWERING*†

	Active Treatment		Control Treatment	
	CHF	No. Randomized	CHF	No. Randomized
Oslo	0	406	1	379
Veterans Administration Study I (VA I)	0	68	4	63
Veterans Administration Study II (VA II)	0	186	11	194
Australian National Blood Pressure Study (ANBPS)	3	1721	3	1706
US Public Health Service (USPHS)	0	193	2	196
Systolic Hypertension in the Elderly Program (SHEP)	56	2365	109	2371
Swedish Trial in Older Patients with Hypertension (STOP)	19	812	39	815
European Working Party on High Blood Pressure in the Elderly (EWPHE)	7	416	17	424
Coope and Warrender	22	419	36	465

Hypertension-Stroke Cooperative Study Group (HSCSG)	0	233	6	219
Wolf	2	45	8	42
Carter	3	50	4	49
Total: All Trials	112	6914	240	6923

Relative risk 0.48—Treatment:control; 95% confidence interval—0.38, 0.59

* Not recorded in HDFP, MRC and MRC in Elderly.

† *A reduction of 52% in the occurrence of congestive heart failure (CHF) in treated compared to control subjects was noted in these controlled, randomized hypertension treatment trials.*

From: Moser M, Hebert P. *J Am Coll Cardiol.* 1996;27:1214.

16

TABLE 16.4 — EFFECTS OF THERAPY IN OLDER HYPERTENSIVE PATIENTS

	CLINICAL TRIAL NAME							
	Australian	EWPHE	C & W	STOP	MRC	SHEP	HDFP	Syst Eur
Number of patients	582	840	884	1,627	4,396	4,736	2,374	4,695
Age range (years)	60-69	>60	60-79	70-84	65-74	60-≥80	60-69	>60
Mean blood pressure at entry, mm Hg	165/101	182/101	197/100	195/102	185/91	170/77	170/101	174/86
Percent Reduction in Events in Treated Compared to Controls								
Stroke	33	36	42*	47*	25*	33*	44*	42*
CAD	18	20	+.03	13†	19	27*	15*	30
CHF	—	22	32	51*	—	55*	—	29
All CVD	31	29*	24*	40*	17*	32*	16*	31*

Abbreviations: EWPHE, European Working Party on High Blood Pressure in the Elderly; C & W, Coope and Warrender; STOP, Swedish Trial in Older Patients with Hypertension; MRC, Medical Research Council Study; SHEP, Systolic Hypertension in the Elderly Program; HDFP, Hypertension Detection and Follow-up Program; Syst Eur, European Trial on Isolated Systolic Hypertension in the Elderly; CAD, Coronary artery disease; CHF, Congestive heart failure; CVD, Cerebrovascular disease.

* Statistically significant.
† Myocardial infarction only; sudden deaths decreased from 13 to 4.

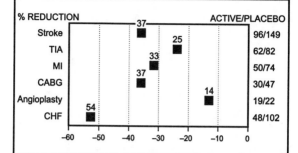

FIGURE 16.3 — SHEP: NONFATAL EVENTS

% REDUCTION   ACTIVE/PLACEBO

Event	% Reduction	Active/Placebo
Stroke	37	96/149
TIA	25	62/82
MI	33	50/74
CABG	37	30/47
Angioplasty	14	19/22
CHF	54	48/102

Abbreviations: TIA, transient ischemic attack; MI, myocardial infarction; CABG, coronary artery bypass graft; CHF, congestive heart failure.

Percent reduction in nonfatal events in the Systolic Hypertension in the Elderly Program (SHEP).

SHEP Study Cooperative Research Group. *JAMA*. 1991;265: 3255-3264.

physicians may not be aware of the major benefits of therapy and may not be implementing therapy early enough or pursuing it vigorously enough to achieve good results. Patient adherence to therapy can be increased by following some of the suggestions below.

With the advent of newer agents that may act more physiologically or may act on other risk factors, we may be able to improve the results of treatment even more dramatically. The important point to remember is that if you are going to achieve results as good as or better than those achieved in the clinical trials, careful attention must be paid to:

- Keeping the regimen as simple as possible
- Keeping expense of treatment at a reasonable level
- Setting a goal of normotensive levels (< 140/ 90 mm Hg) and adhering to this goal as closely as possible.

16

This may not always be easy to achieve in elderly patients, but in the majority of patients, it is possible.

17 Selected Readings

Diagnosis

Pickering TG, Devereux RB. Ambulatory monitoring of blood pressure as a predictor of cardiovascular risk. *Am Heart J.* 1987;114: 925-928.

Joint National Committee on Detection, Evaluation and Treatment of High Blood Pressure. Fifth Report of the Joint National Committee on Detection, Evaluation and Treatment of High Blood Pressure (JNC-V). *Arch Intern Med.* 1993;153:154-183.

Joint National Committee on Detection, Evaluation and Treatment of High Blood Pressure. Sixth Report of the Joint National Committee on Detection, Evaluation and Treatment of High Blood Pressure (JNC-VI). *Arch Intern Med.* In press.

Julius S, Mejia A, Jones K, et al. "White coat" versus "systemic" borderline hypertension in Tecumseh Study. *Hypertension.* 1990;16:617-623.

Levy D, Anderson KM, Savage DD, et al. Echocardiographically detected left ventricular hypertrophy: prevalence and risk factors: the Framingham Heart Study. *Ann Intern Med.* 1988;108:7-13.

Lifestyle/Nonpharmacological Interventions

Alderman MH, Madhavan S, Cohen H, Sealey JE, Laragh JH. Low urinary sodium is associated with greater risk of myocardial infarction among treated hypertensive men. *Hypertension.* 1995;25:1144-1152.

Cutler JA, Follmann D, Elliott P, Suh I. An overview of randomized trials of sodium reduction and blood pressure. *Hypertension.* 1991;17(suppl 1):1-27–1-33.

Hypertension Prevention Trial Research Group. The Hypertension Prevention Trial: three-year effects of dietary changes on blood pressure. *Arch Intern Med.* 1990;150:153-162.

Langford HG, Davis BR, Blaufox MD, et al. Effect of drug and diet treatment of mild hypertension on diastolic blood pressure. *Hypertension.* 1991;17:210-217.

17

Linas SL. The role of potassium in the pathogenesis and treatment of hypertension. *Kidney Int*. 1991;38:771-786.

Stamler R, Stamler J, Gosch FC, et al. Primary prevention of hypertension by nutritional-hygienic means: final report of a randomized, controlled trial. *JAMA*. 1989;262:1801-1807.

Stamler R, Stamler J, Grimm R, et al. Nutritional therapy for high blood pressure: final report of a four-year randomized controlled trial—the Hypertension Control Program. *JAMA*. 1987;257:1484-1491.

Subcommittee on Nonpharmacologic Therapy of the 1984 Joint National Committee on Detection, Evaluation and Treatment of High Blood Pressure. Nonpharmacological approaches to the control of high blood pressure. *Hypertension*. 1986;8:444-467.

Trials of Hypertension Prevention Collaborative Research Group. The effects of nonpharmacologic interventions of blood pressure of persons with high normal levels: results of the Trials of Hypertension Prevention, Phase I. *JAMA*. 1992;267:1213-1220.

World Hypertension League. Alcohol and hypertension—implications for management: a consensus statement by the World Hypertension League. *J Hum Hypertens*. 1991;5:1854-1856.

Pharmacologic Therapy

Eisen SA, Miller DK, Woodward RS, Spitznagel E, Przybeck TR. The effect of prescribed daily dose frequency on patient medication compliance. *Arch Intern Med*. 1990;150:1881-1884.

Furberg C. Final results of the Multicenter Isradipine Diuretic Atherosclerosis Study (MIDAS). Presented at the International Society of Hypertension Meeting. March 22, 1994. Melbourne, Australia.

Gifford RW Jr. Management of hypertensive crises. *JAMA*. 1991;266:829-835.

Gurwitz GH, Bohn RL, Glynn RJ, Monane M, Mogun H, Avorn J. Antihypertensive drug therapy and the initiation of treatment for diabetes mellitus. *Ann Intern Med*. 1993;118:273-278.

Hypertension Detection and Follow-up Program Cooperative Group. Five-year findings of the Hypertension Detection and Follow-up Program (HDFP), 1: reduction in mortality of persons with high blood pressure, including mild hypertension. *JAMA*. 1979;242:2562-2571.

Joint National Committee on Detection, Evaluation and Treatment of High Blood Pressure. Fifth Report of the Joint National Committee on Detection, Evaluation and Treatment of High Blood Pressure (JNC-V). *Arch Intern Med.* 1993;153:154-183.

Joint National Committee on Detection, Evaluation and Treatment of High BLood Pressure. Sixth Report of the Joint National Committee on Detection, Evaluation and Treatment of High Blood Pressure (JNC-VI). *Arch Intern Med.* In press.

Materson BJ, Reda DJ, Cushman WC, et al. Single-drug therapy for hypertension in men: a comparison of six antihypertensive agents with placebo: results of a Department of Veterans Affairs Cooperative Study. *N Engl J Med.* 1993;328:914-921.

Materson BJ, Reda DJ, Williams D. Lessons from combination therapy in Veterans Affairs Studies. Department of Veterans Affairs Cooperative Study Group on antihypertensive agents. *Am J Hypertens.* 1996;9(Pt 2):187S-191S.

Moser M. Antihypertensive medications: relative efficacy and adverse reactions. *J Hypertens.* 1990;8(suppl 2):S9-S16.

Moser M. Can the cost of care be contained and quality of care maintained in the management of hypertension? *Arch Intern Med.* 1994;154:1665-1672.

Moser M. Current hypertension management: separating fact from fiction. *Cleve Clin J Med.* 1993;60:27-37.

Moser M, Ross H. The treatment of hypertension in diabetic patients. *Diabetes Care.* 1993;16:542-547.

Multiple Risk Factor Intervention Trial Research Group. Mortality rates after 10.5 years for participants in the Multiple Risk Factor Intervention Trial (MRFIT): findings related to a prior hypotheses of the trial. *JAMA.* 1990;263:1795-1801.

National High Blood Pressure Education Program Working Group on high blood pressure in pregnancy. Working Group Report on high blood pressure in pregnancy. *Am J Obstet Gynecol.* 1990; 163:1689-1712.

Neaton JD, Grimm RH Jr, Prineas RJ, et al. Treatment of Mild Hypertension Study (TOMHS): final results. *JAMA.* 1993;270:713-724.

Papademetriou V, Burris JF, Notargiacomo A, et al. Thiazide therapy is not a cause of arrhythmia in patients with systemic hypertension. *Arch Intern Med.* 1988;148:1272-1276.

17

Pollare T, Lithell H, Berne C. A comparison of the effects of hydrochlorothiazide and captopril on glucose and lipid metabolism in patients with hypertension. *N Engl J Med*. 1989;321:868.

Tarazi RC, Dustan HP, Frohlich ED. Long-term thiazide therapy in essential hypertension: evidence for persistent alteration in plasma volume and renin activity. *Circulation*. 1970;41:709-717.

■ Results of Therapy

Hebert PR, Moser M, Mayer J, Hennekens CH. Recent evidence on drug therapy of mild to moderate hypertension and decreased risk of coronary heart disease. *Arch Intern Med*. 1993;153:578-581.

Moser M, Hebert P. An overview of the meta-analyses of the hypertension treatment trials. *Arch Intern Med*. 1991;151: 1277-1279.

Moser M, Hebert P. Prevention of disease progression, left ventricular hypertrophy and congestive heart failure in the hypertension treatment trials. *J Am Coll Cardiol*. 1996;27:1214-1218.

Moser M. Angiotensin converting enzyme inhibitors, angiotensin II receptor antagonists and calcium channel blocking agents. A review of potential benefits and possible adverse reactions. *J Am Coll Cardiol*. 1997;29:1414-1421.

■ Treatment of the Elderly

Curb JD, Pressel SL, Cutler JA, et al. Effect of diuretic-based antihypertensive treatment on cardiovascular disease risk in older diabetic patients with isolated systolic hypertension. Systolic Hypertension in the Elderly Program Cooperative Research Group. *JAMA*. 1996;276:1886-1892.

Dahlof B, Lundholm L, Hansson L, Schersten B, Ekbom T, Wester P. Morbidity and mortality in the Swedish Trial in Older Patients with Hypertension (STOP-Hypertension). *Lancet*. 1991;338:1281-1285.

MRC Working Party. Medical Research Council trial of treatment of hypertension in older adults: principal results. *BMJ* . 1992;304: 405-412.

SHEP Cooperative Research Group. Prevention of stroke by antihypertensive drug treatment in older persons with isolated systolic hypertension: final results of the Systolic Hypertension in the Elderly Program (SHEP). *JAMA*. 1991;265:3255-3264.

Staesson JA, Fagard R, Thijs L, et al. Morbidity and mortality in the placebo-controlled trial of Isolated Systolic Hypertension in the Elderly. The Systolic Hypertension-Europe (Syst Eur) Trial. *Lancet*. In press.

Note: Page numbers in *italics* indicate figures;
page numbers followed by t indicate tables.